Pharmacopolitics

STUDIES IN SOCIAL MEDICINE

ALLAN M. BRANDT AND LARRY R. CHURCHILL, *editors*

Pharmacopolitics

**Drug Regulation
in the United States
and Germany**

✦ ————————————————————————

by Arthur A. Daemmrich

THE UNIVERSITY OF NORTH CAROLINA PRESS

Chapel Hill and London

Designed by Gary Gore
Set in Monotype Dante
by Keystone Typesetting, Inc.

The paper in this book meets the guidelines for permanence and durability
of the Committee on Production Guidelines for Book Longevity of the
Council on Library Resources.

Library of Congress Cataloging-in-Publication Data
Daemmrich, Arthur A.
Pharmacopolitics : drug regulation in the United States and Germany /
by Arthur A. Daemmrich.
p. cm. — (Studies in social medicine)
Includes bibliographical references and index.
ISBN 0-8078-2844-0 (cloth: alk. paper)
1. Pharmaceutical policy—United States. 2. Pharmaceutical policy—Germany.
3. Drugs—Law and legislation—United States. 4. Drugs—Law and legislation—
Germany.
[DNLM: 1. Legislation, Drug—Germany. 2. Legislation, Drug—United States.
3. Clinical Trials—Germany. 4. Clinical Trials—United States. 5. Government
Regulation—Germany. 6. Government Regulation—United States.
7. International Cooperation—Germany. 8. International Cooperation—United
States. 9. Pharmaceutical Preparations—Germany. 10. Pharmaceutical
Preparations—United States.
QV 33 AA1 D123p 2004] I. Title: Drug regulation in the United States and
Germany. II. Title. III. Series.
RA401.A3 D34 2004
362.17′82′0973—dc22
2003016296

08 07 06 05 04   5 4 3 2 1

Contents

Preface ix

Abbreviations xiii

1 Introduction: Medicine, Politics, and Governance 1

2 Drug Laws and Therapeutic Cultures 19

3 Clinical Trials from Treatment to Test, 1950–1980 48

4 Clinical Trials as Test and Therapy, 1980–2000 81

5 Configuring the Market as a Testing Site 116

6 Conclusion: International Harmonization and the
Future of Drug Regulation 151

Appendix: Research Methods and Case Study Selection 165

Notes 167

Bibliography 181

Index 199

Figures and Tables

Figures

1	Kennedy signing the 1962 Kefauver-Harris Amendments into law	28
2	FDA protest, 1988	31
3	AIDS cases by year of reporting, 1980–2000	43
4	AMA Registry on Adverse Reactions, 1966	122
5	AkdÄ reporting form, 1964	129
6	FDA Drug Experience Report, 1967	135
7	FDA MEDWatch reporting form, contemporary	139
8	AkdÄ reporting form, contemporary	144

Tables

1	Sites for Therapeutic Cultures	16
2	Case Studies—Market Authorization	17
3	Turning Points in American Drug Regulation	33
4	Turning Points in German Drug Regulation	41
5	ECOG Performance Status	88
6	Therapeutic Cultures	152
7	"The Patient"	154

Preface

"So which country is better?" Physicians, industry insiders, and academic colleagues occasionally posed this challenge while I researched and wrote this book. For a social scientist comparing two political, regulatory, and medical systems, this question can be very hard to answer. Health care seems to have entered a state of permanent crisis in both countries in the past three decades: physicians, hospitals, and insurers complain of impending bankruptcy, patients feel ignored or mistreated, and governments find that every policy change creates a host of new problems. Drug prices go up and the ability of insurers and the insured to pay for drugs declines with each passing year. In both countries, seemingly useless or unsafe medicines seem to come on the market, while apparently life-saving drugs are delayed for years in clinical testing.

Drug regulation is a complex system in which physicians, government regulators, the pharmaceutical industry, and disease-based organizations fight about or, less frequently, collaborate on clinical trials, approval decisions, and the monitoring of side effects. As readers of this book will discover, the institutions that govern this system are nationally and historically specific. Therefore, transferring approaches from one to the other is no easy feat. To eliminate the U.S. Food and Drug Administration, as is proposed on occasion, would leave important needs of ill people and the general public unmet. Likewise, to greatly strengthen federal regulation in Germany would upset a system of local and regional physician authority that historically has addressed the majority of patients' concerns.

For this reason, to focus solely on the question "Which is better?" distracts from understanding the values held by citizens and embodied in governing institutions in each country. The salience of principles and values to debates concerning how illness should be treated, acceptable levels of surveillance by medical authorities and the state, and what kinds of data should be used to make decisions about the market status of pharmaceuticals will only increase in coming years. As I argue in the pages that follow, the relationship of sick people to their medicines has become a crucial aspect of how citizens relate to their governments. These relations will have a major impact on the development of a globally "harmonized" set of rules for drug regulation currently underway. With so many health care needs going unmet—even in wealthy countries like the United States and Germany—learning from past mistakes and accounting for the values of diverse patient populations are crucial to the design of this emerging international system.

This study has benefited enormously from the critical insights of academic colleagues, the support of friends and family members, and the financial backing of several universities and foundations. Sheila Jasanoff guided my graduate education, commented on multiple drafts of this book, and mentored a collaborative network of science studies scholars at Cornell and Harvard. A number of people read and reacted to one or more of the chapters, including Harry Marks, Glenn Sonnedecker, Volker Hess, Alastair Iles, Nick King, and Georg Krücken. Steven Epstein and anonymous reviewers for the University of North Carolina Press provided insightful comments and suggestions on the final manuscript. To the extent that this book offers a reasoned comparative perspective on the relations of medicine and the state in the United States and Germany during the twentieth century, I have these people to thank for it; flaws remaining in the text are my responsibility. I also thank Sian Hunter, Paula Wald, Eric Schramm, and other staff members of the University of North Carolina Press for their excellent work in guiding this book through production.

Research in the United States was greatly helped by John Swann at the Food and Drug Administration and Greg Higby at the American Institute of the History of Pharmacy. In Berlin, Rolf Winau generously arranged an office at the Institut für Geschichte der Medizin. Peter Dilg and Fritz Krafft opened the doors of the Institut für Geschichte der Pharmazie at the University of Marburg to an inquisitive scholar. Likewise, Frances Kelsey at the FDA, Volker Dinnendahl at the Arzneimittelkommission der deutschen Apotheker, Gisbert Selke at the Wissenschaftliches Institut der AOK, Eberhard Baumbauer at the Verband Forschender Arzneimittelhersteller, Barbara Sickmüller at the Bundesverband der Pharmazeutischen Industrie, and Catia Monser, Axel Murswieck, Georges Fülgraf, Ernst Habermann, and Karl Kimbel all allowed me to interview them and provided access to key documents. Karl-Heinz Munter of the Arzneimittelkommission der deutschen Ärzteschaft deserves special mention for his interest in my research and for letting me drive his Jaguar on the Autobahn.

This project would not have been completed without the generous funding of the Cornell Department of Science and Technology Studies, the Berlin Program for Advanced German and European Studies (jointly administered by the Freie Universität Berlin and the Social Science Research Council), the Kennedy School of Government at Harvard University, and the Chemical Heritage Foundation. Through its support for research on the molecular science industries, history of chemistry, and science and technology policy, the Chemical Heritage Foundation has proven itself a stimulating intellectual environment and collegial professional home for the past several years.

Finally, my greatest thanks go to Saiping Tso for her (im)patience, support, and love.

Abbreviations

ACT UP AIDS Coalition to Unleash Power
AkdÄ   Arzneimittelkommission der deutschen Ärzteschaft (Drug Commission of the Federal Chamber of Physicians)
AMA   American Medical Association
BÄK   Bundesärztekammer (Federal Chamber of Physicians)
BfArM   Bundesinstitut für Arzneimittel- und Medizinprodukte (Federal Institute for Pharmaceutical and Medicinal Products)
BGA   Bundesgesundheitsamt (Federal Health Office)
CPMP   Commission on Proprietary Medicinal Products
ECOG   Eastern Cooperative Oncology Group
EMEA   European Agency for the Evaluation of Medicinal Products
EPAR   European Public Assessment Report
FDA   Food and Drug Administration
ICH   International Conference on Harmonisation of Technical Requirements for Registration of Pharmaceuticals for Human Use
ICI   Imperial Chemical Industries
NCI   National Cancer Institute
NDA   New Drug Application
NF   National Formulary
NGO   Non-Governmental Organization
NIH   National Institutes of Health
NKCA   National Kidney Cancer Association
SPD   Social-Democratic Party
TAG   Treatment Action Group
USDA   United States Department of Agriculture
USP   United States Pharmacopoeia

Pharmacopolitics

1 Introduction

Medicine, Politics, and Governance

IN RECENT YEARS, PHARMACEUTICAL DRUGS HAVE become implicated in global politics as never before. Inequitable drug prices, persisting differences in national regulatory approaches, and debates over how to define safety and efficacy for diverse patient populations around the globe now attract an unprecedented degree of attention. The political, financial, and human health stakes have never been higher for patients, manufacturers, government agencies, or the medical profession.

Unlike the conventional terrain of macro-politics where states collide over interests of national security, pharmaceutical politics play out at a level where citizens deal with illness and health and small organizations voice demands for greater representation. The "high" politics that shape relations among countries and determine governance structures at the national and international level now can be found in the "low" arenas of drug regulation and health care delivery. Power and politics are not just found at the level of nations or international agreements, but are wrapped up in seemingly innocuous pharmaceutical drugs and supposedly standardized regimes for verifying their safety and efficacy. Debates over pharma-

1

ceutical drugs in this "low" arena ultimately shape the organization of states, industry, the medical profession, and non-governmental organizations (NGOs).

Recent events offer some striking illustrations of these points. Seeking to reduce the cost of medicines for their citizens, the governments of India, South Africa, Brazil, and other countries have threatened to ignore drug patents and institute compulsory licensing initiatives. Pharmaceutical firms headquartered in the United States and Europe defend drug prices by explaining the expenses accrued during research and testing. Between 6,000 and 10,000 compounds are synthesized in the laboratory for each drug that ultimately enters the marketplace. During 2001, pharmaceutical companies spent an average of 17 percent of sales on research and development, an outlay of $30 billion in the United States and $12 billion in Europe. According to industry-sponsored surveys, getting a new drug from the laboratory to patients requires companies to invest $800 million over the course of ten to twelve years.[1] As evidence for current pricing patterns and enforcing strict patent laws, these facts nevertheless fall on deaf ears when government officials and activists attack firms for failing to meet the health care needs of patients in developing countries. In response, the industry has slashed prices—most notably for AIDS drugs—and has increased efforts to help poor nations improve their health care systems.[2]

Drawing a link among disease, poverty, and terrorism, U.S. President Bush recently proposed an "Emergency Plan for AIDS Relief" to help an estimated thirty million Africans suffering from the illness. In his 2003 State of the Union address, Bush asked for $10 billion in new funds so that "this nation can lead the world in sparing innocent people from a plague of nature." Much of this new support would underwrite the purchase and delivery of anti-retroviral drugs, which Bush noted had declined in price from $12,000 to under $300 per year of treatment. A $15 billion initiative took shape during spring 2003; among other goals, the Bush administration plans to use these funds to make therapeutic drugs available to two million Africans with HIV. Not coincidentally, Bush's speech turned next to national security: "And this nation is leading the world in confronting and defeating the man-made evil of international terrorism."[3]

In the context of security concerns, Bayer was forced to renegotiate the price and availability of its antibiotic Ciproflaxin following anthrax attacks in the fall of 2001.[4] An uproar concerning bioterrorist threats brought shifts in the relationship among government, industry, and the public to the fore. When Tom Brokaw of NBC Nightly News held up a container of the pills and stated, "In Cipro we trust," he drew attention to the significance of modern biomedicine for national security and the public's trust in governing authorities.[5] Fearing shortages, government officials in Canada and the United States threatened to ignore Bayer's patent rights by licensing generic manufacturers to produce the drug. The company ultimately avoided this scenario by increasing stockpiles and cutting prices.

In both the case of AIDS medicines in developing countries and anthrax treatments in industrialized nations, intellectual property rights and drug prices came under fire for threatening public health and national security. Policy solutions in both settings involved negotiated compromise rather than strict regulation. States that once governed industry sectors through command-and-control mechanisms now negotiate with global companies. Patients who once interacted with issues of drug prices, safety, and availability mediated only through their physicians now are organized as autonomous influential political actors. These developments offer an interesting and exciting vision for the future as power and authority are shared among national governments, multinational companies, and NGOs.

Offering a distinctly technocratic vision for this future, government officials and representatives of the pharmaceutical industry from the United States, the European Union, and Japan have met regularly during the past decade in an attempt to develop uniform standards for clinical trials and regulatory review. They intend to standardize all aspects of drug testing and reduce the costs and time involved in bringing new medicines to the market. Participants in this "International Conference on Harmonization of Technical Requirements for Registration of Pharmaceuticals for Human Use" (ICH) hope to achieve this goal by rationalizing safety and efficacy testing. They expect test results, like the pills themselves, will transfer easily from any one political and medical context to another.

The standardization of medical policies along the spectrum from premarket testing to patient surveillance once drugs are marketed will require the mobilization of multiple actors. It will also require changes in a variety of less visibly political settings. Concerns about representation, drug costs, and access to medical care are not just negotiated in the course of government regulatory decisions, but also during clinical trials and in the doctor-patient relationship. As the examples of AIDS and anthrax illustrate, the extremely contentious issue of drug prices is linked to regulatory demands for product safety, scientific debates regarding testing methods, and moral concerns with patients' rights. These features of national medical politics are likely to resist global standardization.

Therapeutic Cultures in the United States and Germany

Advances in medicine, the emergence and persistence of intractable diseases, high-profile drug disasters, and even low-profile medical errors all fuel debates among the principal actors in medical politics. Throughout this book, I advance the concept of *therapeutic cultures* as shorthand for relationships among the state (including legislatures and regulatory agencies), the pharmaceutical industry, the medical profession, and disease-based organizations. These actors frequently offer rival visions for health care with profound implications for the organization of modern societies. Competition over who can best speak for "the patient" was fundamental to the assertion of authority in this arena. While the direct claims made by patients regarding the impact of disease and the appropriateness of competing treatments have reached broader audiences in recent years, for the bulk of the twentieth century, patients did not speak directly in health care policy. Instead, professional groups and government agencies competed for the authority to represent them. As we shall see, differences between therapeutic cultures in the United States and Germany, the two countries on which this book focuses, resulted in very different choices for regulatory structures and produced different therapeutic orientations to their national polities.

Therapeutic cultures, as I employ the term, refers specifically to the historical evolution of a distinctive set of institutionalized relationships among the state, industry, physicians, and disease-based organizations. I argue throughout this book that the United States and Germany have put into place two different sets of these institutional relations through incremental historical processes. Their therapeutic cultures share a close interface with broader political and cultural beliefs and practices that are intriguingly similar and different between the two countries. Since 1950, citizens of both West Germany and the United States have experienced stable forms of democratic governance, remarkable advances in medical technologies, capitalist economies that support free trade, and government involvement in medicine through research support and regulation of the pharmaceutical market.

These similarities are offset by contrasts in their health insurance arrangements, access of patients to the political process, the authority wielded by physicians, and social insurance systems. For example, health care in the United States is generally seen as a private good associated with individual choice and the availability of "menus" for insurance, thereby rationing care by price. In Germany, by contrast, health care is seen primarily as a right or entitlement. It serves as an instrument of broader social justice, and rationing, if at all, is controlled by providers on a local and individual level.

This institutionalist perspective on politics and culture sheds light on the relation between broader cultural beliefs and practices on the one hand and institutional relations and policy outcomes on the other. The case of pharmaceutical regulation and medical care shows that there is no simple causal relationship between these two domains: we cannot argue that *because* Germany has cultural belief X, it has institutions x; or alternatively, *because* the United

States has institutions y, it has cultural belief Y. Yet in key instances, the cultural patterns exhibited in medical care in Germany differ from those of the United States *in the same way* that their institutions differ.[6] In action—not least in the definition of "the patient," care for the ill, and formal medical policy—there are tight reciprocal relationships between cultures and institutions.

The concept of therapeutic cultures helps to untangle some of these connections and draws attention to important contrasts between the United States and Germany. Differences between the two countries are especially meaningful in light of similarities in their official requirements for drug safety and efficacy, as well as their overarching similarities in medical care. Therapeutic cultures are active in three primary arenas: legislative / regulatory mandates, scientific testing in clinical trials, and oversight of adverse drug reactions. Because of their different therapeutic cultures, the distribution of authority among the quartet of actors in medical policy has shifted frequently in the United States, but remained comparatively stable in Germany. In one key feature of medical policy, American regulators delineated a strict boundary between premarket testing and market approval, whereas their German counterparts adopted a more flexible approach that blurred the line between pre- and postmarket oversight. More recently, differences between their therapeutic cultures promoted the emergence of disease-based interest groups targeting regulatory policy in the United States, while few such organizations sought to change regulatory approaches in Germany.

This means of explaining differences between the two countries brings into focus the shifting role of politics in medicine. Instead of viewing regulatory differences as the outcome of variation in state structures, we see that the political challenges posed by medical risks are mediated by a more complex web of relationships among the state and the other major participants in health care delivery—including, most significantly, the medical profession. The United States and Germany have some similar and some different ways of interrelating patient needs with pharmaceutical research and testing, medical care, and government regulation. In both countries, knowledge production and decision-making authority are distributed across a network of key actors including industry, the medical profession, government agencies, and disease-based organizations. Yet differences in the relationships among the actors account for the fact that drug testing and scientific procedures have become politicized in the United States, but not in Germany.

Comparing the United States and Germany

The primary purpose of this book is to compare drug regulation in the United States and Germany between 1950 and the present. For the period between 1950 and 1990, "Germany" refers explicitly to the Federal Republic of Germany, or West Germany. The German Democratic Republic (DDR) had a unique set of political and structural constraints on medicine and a radically different relationship between the state and civil society, making it inappropriate for this study. During the past decade, a reunited Germany has gradually integrated key features of its government with the European Union. For that reason, the comparison is expanded in Chapter 4 to encompass European-level regulations and clinical testing.

Throughout the book, I explore several puzzling differences between the United States and Germany. First, government officials in the United States closely control the production of information about the safety and efficacy of new medicines, whereas the medical profession has retained greater autonomy to design and oversee clinical testing in Germany. Second, a strict division between testing and marketing prevails in the United States, while German institutions follow a more flexible regime regarding pre- and postmarket regulatory oversight. Third, patients in the United States increasingly challenge expert risk assessments and demand access to drugs, even in early stages of clinical trials. A comparable politics of patient identity and access to medicines is strikingly absent in Germany, where professional associations continue to operate as intermediaries between citizens and the state.

While important in their own right, these differences become even more interesting in light of major similarities and often-subtle contrasts between the principal actors in medical policy and politics in the two countries. Multinational firms headquartered in each country develop most new pharmaceuticals, but frequently market different drugs in each nation. Drugs intended for both countries undergo distinctive tests in each of them. Physicians are accorded a high status and have well-organized political representation in both countries; however, their influence on the government and authority to speak for patients differ. Analogous networks in the two countries pass judgment on the market status of a new drug, yet their decisions vary to a surprising degree. These same networks of government officials, physicians, company officials, and patients monitor approved drugs in each country, but they employ different mechanisms for market surveillance and react differently to side effects. More generally, the United States and Germany developed different regulatory systems during the twentieth century, despite similar citizen pressure to ensure product safety and industry lobbying to reduce barriers to market entry.

Government

Both the United States and Germany since 1950 have had stable, democratically elected governments, although they exhibit different forms of representation, legislation, and regulation. Government authority in both countries is circumscribed by a constitution (termed the Grundgesetz, or basic law, in Germany) that delineates federal and state powers. Even though the United States is a representative democracy and Germany a parliamentary democracy, both have a tripartite division of power among executive, legislative, and judicial branches. Of all liberal-democratic countries, citizens in the United States and Germany most closely share the belief that strict limits should be placed on government authority, albeit for different reasons. The United States has a long tradition of balancing individual freedom against state interests. Citizens hold powers not expressly granted to the government, and vociferously defend their rights through political protest and legal action. For Germany, the Nazi dictatorship sharply illustrated that the concentration of power within a single political party with a charismatic leader could lead to destructive and inhuman policies. Consequently, the Grundgesetz strengthened federalism and placed a strong emphasis on the rule of law.

The executive branch differs in important ways between these two countries. American presidents are chosen during an independent election every four years and play a significant role in setting policy agendas, advancing legislative initiatives, and overseeing regulatory action. In Germany, the Bundeskanzler is elected by parliament, generally as head of the majority party. The Bundeskanzler's ability to shape policy agendas is constrained by party politics and the need to enter political coalitions with other parties to establish a parliamentary majority. Most new laws are proposed by the ruling coalition, not by individual parliamentary representatives. This gives the Bundeskanzler a larger role in crafting legislation than typically is held by the American president.

The U.S. legislature is divided between the House of Representatives and the Senate; both must ratify legislation in order for it to become law. Congress plays an important role as a watchdog over the execution of laws. Investigative committees and congressional hearings frequently examine issues of political concern soon after they arise. Germany also has a bicameral parliament; the Bundestag represents public interests, while the upper house, the Bundesrat, represents the states (Länder). The Bundesrat votes on legislation that would impact the division of power between the federal government and the Länder. It can delay, but not veto, other legislation. Whereas the public elects both the American House and Senate, German citizens elect only representatives in the Bundestag. Bundesrat membership is composed solely of representatives from the Länder. According to some analysts, the German parliament has been very constrained in its oversight of how laws are executed and in its responses to new policy concerns.[7]

Each country makes provisions for judicial review of new laws and regulations. The U.S. Supreme Court early on asserted its constitutional authority to declare legislative acts invalid or unconstitutional. It nevertheless serves primarily as the country's highest court of appeals, not as a specialized court. In the aftermath of the Nazi dictatorship, the German system was constructed with a Federal Constitutional Court that resolves disputes among government authorities and protects the basic rights of citizens. More generally, Germany employs a continental law system under which judges interpret codified laws. The United States, by contrast, bases legal decisions on case law (precedent) and trial by peer juries.

Restrictive tort laws limit lawsuits in Germany and claims against manufacturers such as drug companies rarely produce large settlements. Scientific and medical experts are generally called as court-appointed witnesses in these and other cases, not as experts for the prosecution or defense. In contrast, American tort law intentionally sets a low barrier to legal access for citizens and different expert witnesses can testify for each side of a case. Despite claims that U.S. tort law impedes innovation and is extremely costly to manufacturers, liability is not uniform across product categories. Contraceptives, vaccines, and drugs taken during pregnancy are especially subject to liability claims in the United States. Thus three products, the Dalkon Shield contraceptive, Bendectin (a treatment for pregnancy-related nausea), and silicon breast implants have composed the majority of liability litigation in the health care sector during the past three decades.[8]

Since World War II, the United States and Germany have experienced a similar growth in government bureaucracies. New and expanded agencies faced similar pressures to draw upon scientific and medical expertise when making decisions.[9] Regulatory agencies overseeing the pharmaceutical industry in the two countries develop and maintain their authority in similar ways by demanding premarket testing and formal application for market approval. New drugs achieve marketable status only if the manufacturer complies with government guidelines for testing and provides authorities with evidence of their safety and efficacy. In both countries, drug companies must pay for clinical trials, oversee the clinics that test drugs, and then submit formal results to the government. Likewise, regulatory agencies in both countries assess "user fees" to companies that want to expedite the review process.

The Pharmaceutical Industry

Both nations have seen matching growth in multinational drug firms and industry investments in research, advertising, and lobbying. Serving as major employers and contributors to the economy, pharmaceutical companies also provide a vital public service by marketing new therapies to treat disease. The combined R&D investment in the United States by pharmaceutical firms was $32 billion in 2002.[10] In the same year, drug companies invested $3 billion on R&D in Germany.[11] Worldwide, the United States receives 36 percent of pharmaceutical R&D investments, while Germany comes in third (after Japan) at 10 percent. The pharmaceutical industry accounts for over 18 percent of all corporate-sponsored research and employs nearly 5 percent of all research scientists and engineers.[12]

As a number of critics have recently noted, massive R&D investments are coupled to aggressive advertising. For this and other reasons, both countries have undergone a blossoming in "drug culture" as their citizens expect and even demand quick fixes for a wide variety of diseases, disorders, and discomforts. Speaking mostly about Americans, the commentator Andrew Sullivan recently noted, "We are taking advantage of living in the 21st century and medicating ourselves to the gills."[13] Germans have also noted and criticized extremely widespread use of pharmaceuticals in their country. People in the two countries spend roughly the same amount for prescription drugs each year. Thus in 1997, per capita spending on pharmaceuticals in the United States was $319, while Germans spent the equivalent of $294 per person on medications.[14]

In terms of the number of pharmaceutical products available, Germany is a global leader with some 2,500 approved active substances (equating to 8,900 drug products), compared to 1,200 (6,000 products) available in the United States.[15] Measured by sales, the United States has the world's largest drug market, followed closely by the European Union. Together, they now account for over 65 percent of annual drug purchases worldwide. Although not always reflected in drug prices, the pharmaceutical market is extremely competitive and sales are distributed across a large number of companies. Over the last decade, the combined worldwide market share of the top thirty pharmaceutical and biotechnology firms has held steady at just over 50 percent. Even the largest of these companies holds patents on only 6.5 percent of the pharmaceutical drugs approved in the United States.[16] Sales are likewise distributed across many firms; Pfizer, the current industry leader, captured just 7.3 percent of worldwide drug sales in 2002.[17]

While it made sense to speak of an "American" or "German" pharmaceutical company as recently as a decade ago, mergers and greater cross-national R&D investments have since rendered these categories less significant. Thus reports of Abbott Laboratories' performance now incorporate BASF's drug business. Likewise, the 1999 creation of Aventis signaled a merger of Hoechst and Rhône-Poulenc, formerly venerable independent German and French firms. These and other pharmaceutical companies all seek to market their medicines across the globe and work with physicians in a variety of settings to meet regulatory demands.

Physicians and Patients

German medical practitioners tap into a long history as a guild-based profession. During a period of intense political ferment in the 1840s, physicians played a significant role in an effort to establish a constitutional democracy for the emerging German nation.[18] Following the failed 1848 revolution, physicians avoided further confrontations with the Prussian-led government by adopting self-regulatory initiatives and agreeing to govern key features of the health care sector in collaboration with government ministers. The profession's retreat from overt political engagement therefore was coupled to its expanded authority over the medical domain. Physicians determined membership criteria for the profession, gained a monopoly to speak for "the patient" in political settings, and had the authority to define drug safety and oversee the use of pharmaceutical drugs. To this day, these features continue to make the medical profession a major actor in medical policy and politics. The fact that twentieth-century regulations governing pharmaceutical drug safety and efficacy assigned a great deal of authority to physicians illustrates a continuation of this historical pattern.

Nineteenth-century American physicians exercised similar controls over membership in the profession, spoke for their patients in political settings, and oversaw drugs on the market.[19] Unlike the German Federal Chamber of Physicians (Bundesärztekammer), the American Medical Association (AMA) progressively lost membership, from a peak near 70 percent of physicians in the mid-1930s to only roughly 35 percent today.[20] When the Food and Drug Administration (FDA) expanded its authority through a sequence of legislative and regulatory initiatives, physicians' authority to define drug safety and ability to control the use of pharmaceuticals declined. Likewise, the emergence of disease-based interest groups as major social and political organizations has undercut the medical profession's mandate to speak for "the patient." While the principal actors in American medical politics appear identical to Germany's, different voices are heard and a different set of concerns come to the fore. No one group can easily claim a monopoly to represent patients in political settings. Pharmaceutical drug regulations in the United States thus are associated with significant renegotiation of authority among the key actors in medical policy.

The methods employed to test new drugs and the procedures followed to verify their safety and efficacy consequently differ between the United States and Germany in important ways. More subtly, but far more significantly, the location of authority to define "safety" and "efficacy" varies. Whereas the German system relies heavily on the medical profession to define the pre- and postmarket status of a drug and oversee standards for clinical testing, the United States has allocated greater authority to government regulators. While American physicians serve as expert consultants to regulatory authorities, the German medical profession itself serves as an authoritative intermediary between patients and the industry. As a result, the American Food and Drug Administration plays a far greater role in all aspects of drug testing and market surveillance than its contemporary counterpart, the Bundesinstitut für Arzneimittel- und Medizinprodukte, in Germany.

Networks in Science, Technology, and Medicine

Therapeutic cultures arise from networks of actors that produce regulatory policy, determine testing standards, and ultimately decide on market access for new drugs. The principal actors in medical policy (regulatory agencies, physicians, pharmaceutical companies, disease-based organizations) form a rather fluid and flexible network that sustains intense debates and very serious differences of opinion. Underpinning their positions, each of these actors draws upon smaller and tighter networks to articulate policy positions concerning medical issues. Like in other networks mapped by sociologists and historians, information flows unevenly, certain points are connected to others more strongly, the "most legitimate spokespersons" change over time, and links are modified during controversies.[21] Stable networks and standardized procedures make it possible for information, ideas, and people to move from one place to another without drawing attention to the social features and assumptions that link any two nodes together.[22] During moments of controversy, however, the stabilizing forces themselves become contentious and connections break down as actors try to extend their individual authority.[23] Each then seeks to become an obligatory "point of passage" for decisions that, for example, certify a new drug as safe and efficacious.

Scientific knowledge is established, assimilated, and transmitted through networks of social trust and authority, rather than by radical skeptical testing as depicted in its dominant public image. Likewise, medical knowledge accumulates less through aggressive falsification than through the gradual widening of networks of practice and dissemination. These social aspects rarely are visible because once facts are accepted, the informal inferences, human judgments, and social, political, and financial features of a network that are integral to the research process disappear from public view.[24]

A dominant technological product, such as a blockbuster drug that outsells its competitors, is not always chosen for its technical superiority alone. Instead, a variety of social factors and informal judgments help determine technological "winners."[25] Similarly, proving drug safety and efficacy involves a body of informal practices and testing methods, no matter how hard regulators and practitioners seek to follow a standardized testing regime. Clinical trials are loci for social, ethical, and even moral debates about appropriate therapies, just as they serve to reinforce social roles for patients and physicians. As a result, the testing methods and results are often very controversial.

Of course, scientific and medical debates mostly do reach closure. Contrary to conventional belief, however, closure is rarely achieved through additional laboratory or clinical testing alone. One reason for this relates to the difficulty of deciding what counts as a proper replication of a test during a controversy. In clinical trials, for example, questions may arise over whether a new series of trials were run in the same way as earlier tests. Did the organizers follow the same approach in diagnosing participants? Did unsuccessful trials follow the same dosage regimen as successful ones? Since an infinite number of these technical questions can be used to question the results of a trial, scientists and physicians face serious challenges in achieving consensus on therapeutic approaches. Debates over the results of clinical trials get tangled up with debates over the adequacy of methods used in the tests. As a result, further testing and additional evidence alone cannot resolve such debates.[26]

Closure to debates appears to come through changes in wider social and institutional commitments. In effect, it takes a network of credible colleagues and institutional support to end a controversy. As we shall see, controversies over drug safety and efficacy often turned into disputes over testing methods themselves. Closure was reached by different mechanisms in the two countries; in the United States, the FDA used its full regulatory authority to end disputes, while in Germany, physicians invoked professional norms and the credibility of their field in order to reach consensus.

To a surprising degree, the networks involved in medical policy differ between countries. In the case of the United States and Germany, even though similar actors are represented in the networks, the distribution of authority and control differs between them in important ways.[27] The primacy of any one node in the network shifted frequently in the United States, allowing for relatively rapid accommodation of new technologies and new social movements that represent patients. The German network instead encouraged continuity over change, thereby limiting policy interventions while favoring committed interests and political stability. The behavior of individual actors and the network's overall stability thus reflect each country's unique therapeutic culture.

Science, Policy, and the State

Clinical trials, and the pharmaceutical sciences more generally, serve instrumental purposes in policy decisions. Societal demands for safe medicines have promoted massive growth of scientific research and product testing during the past century. Despite national variation in research, including clinical trials, decision makers in all countries face a similar "risk" quandary concerning medicinal drugs. If they grant market access to a pharmaceutical later shown to cause side effects, they are criticized for failing to protect the public. Conversely, if they withhold approval of a medicine that cures disease or prolongs life, they are criticized for excessive precaution. To borrow a phrase from risk analyst Jonathan Wiener, efforts to protect patients from dangerous medicines produce "iatrogenic [care-induced] risks of risk management."[28] Likewise, other critics have asserted that regulations often run counter to the public interest by limiting competition among firms and orienting innovation to areas that may not benefit the majority of patients.[29]

Models from political science that seek to explain the role of science in these sorts of policy decisions have often depicted a one-way relationship, summarized most easily as "speaking truth to power."[30] According to this archetype, experts can be placed on a spectrum ranging from scientists, who possess pure knowledge, to politicians, who embody decision-making authority. Scientists provide clear answers to government officials on military, environmental, and medical policy questions.[31]

Empirical research on medical, environmental, and other areas of science and technology policy, however, do not support these archetypes. As it turns out, successful real-world applications often require more than laboratory testing of scientific or medical theories. Sheila Jasanoff, who introduced the term "regulatory science" into widespread use, therefore suggests, "When knowledge is uncertain or ambiguous, as is often the case in science bearing on policy, facts alone are inadequate to compel a choice. Any selection inevitably blends scientific with policy considerations, and policymakers accordingly are forced to look beyond science to legitimate their preferred reading of the evidence."[32] In clinical trials, for example, we find that the science itself necessarily incorporates political dimensions, including choices about representation, and standards of accountability that can influence the outcomes.

Trial results often remain open to political and medical contestation; in the course of a debate over the safety or efficacy of a specific treatment, participants do not separate "political" arguments from "scientific" ones. Questions about the validity of science carried out for regulatory purposes become particularly salient when decision makers seek to predict future outcomes. Thus regulators trying to evaluate whether or not a drug will produce side effects on the open market have to consider the institutional contexts in which the trials were conducted and weigh the likely public responses to their decisions.

Greater awareness of the decision-making dilemma between approving a drug later shown to cause side effects and withholding a beneficial and potentially life-saving therapy has weakened the assumption that scientific or medical research alone can develop predictive tools for public policy.[33] In a number of important areas, the lay public itself has reshaped what counts as scientific evidence, in addition to more predictable demands for greater representation and participation. Efforts spearheaded by AIDS patients to speed drug approvals, for example, also had the outcome of loosening state control over clinical trials and changing the power relationship between physicians and patients. These activists mobilized their own experts to support alternative views of disease origins and dissemination. They also demanded changes in trial protocols and revisions to entry criteria.[34]

More generally, patients, consumers, and social activists not supported by traditional organizations have joined to articulate demands in local, regional, and national arenas. These interest groups employ a wide variety of strategies to gain access to government decisions. In the United States, traditional professional groups like the American Medical Association are structured to match the federal system, thereby gaining policy input at levels ranging from local licensing boards to national politics.[35] New groups, such as AIDS activists, often concentrate on a single issue, which they raise in forums ranging from public protests to congressional hearings. Public readiness to organize new political groups and the openness of the political system to their demands promotes rapid policy response to emerging issues. At the same time, it can lead to very visible conflicts when competing interests clash.

In contrast, associations representing business, professions, churches, and other interests share authority with the decentralized German state.[36] Formally designated interest associations are included within the process of government decision making and help implement new policies. As such, they are officially recognized by the state not just as intermediaries between government officials and the public, but as associations on equal footing with state agencies. Associations do more than lobby the state on behalf of their membership; they also provide expert advice and get involved in both the formulation and implementation of public policy. Since peak associations work so closely with the state, radical changes and sudden policy innovations are relatively infrequent. Incremental changes result from stable compromises between business and the government.[37] Public confrontations between associations and the state are rare in Germany, and decisions about pharmaceutical and environmental regulations, changes to the health care system, and other potentially volatile issues generally are negotiated in a quiet, seemingly apolitical manner.

National-level differences of this sort have gained particular saliency in light of regulatory harmonization both within the European Union and among the United States, Europe, and other countries. Proponents of international regimes argue that abolishing trade barriers, standardizing premarket testing regimes, and harmonizing regulatory oversight will reduce differences among national institutions, promote greater industrial efficiency, and bring cures to patients sooner. As we shall see, the European Union and the emerging international regime for drug regulation both must account for persisting national differences in therapeutic cultures.

For Germany, European integration has taken place concurrently with internal integration of East and West following the 1990 unification. Germany's willingness, even eagerness, to give up sovereign power at a time of national expansion surprised those analysts who predicted a less harmonious outcome. In many ways, Germans have adopted an international and collective identity that promotes broader interest representation and new norms for power relations.[38] Tensions nevertheless remain regarding the status of Germany within Europe, especially since German trade unions and NGOs frequently raise concerns about employment and the environment.

For the United States, participation in international agreements is a highly politicized two-edged sword. Many analysts, activists, and corporate strategists welcome the potential for regulatory harmonization to reduce burdens on industry and speed medicines to the market. On the other hand, critics warn that agreements to date have decreased product safety, weakened regulatory oversight, and led to a loss of jobs. In the environmental arena, the United States seems increasingly willing to forgo global accords and forge its own path. Likewise, risk assessment policies for genetically modified foods, chemicals, and other industrial products more commonly exhibit "American exceptionalism" than harmonization with other countries.[39] The United States nevertheless is an active participant in efforts to unify pre-clinical and clinical testing standards. Technical standardization and international harmonization has therefore proceeded apace in this area. These accords will not automatically equate to global drug approvals or international health care policies. Yet they do illustrate the emergence of a loosely coupled system at the global level in which the United States is a significant participant.

Sites for Therapeutic Cultures

The principal actors in medical policy and politics—government regulatory agencies, pharmaceutical companies, the medical profession, and disease-based organizations—interact in distinct political and medical settings. The chapters that follow describe the impact of American and German therapeutic cultures

TABLE 1 / SITES FOR THERAPEUTIC CULTURES

Country	Legal/Regulatory	Laboratory/Clinic	Marketplace
United States	Rapid legislative response to "drug disasters"; centralized regulatory authority at the FDA	Emergence and dominance of quantitative methods; strict boundary between testing and market	Bureaucratic imperative to compartmentalize, group, and quantify; FDA collects data and responds to side effects
Germany	Legislation only after protracted bargaining and compromise; regulatory authority divided across a network of key players	Qualitative testing methods and communal norms dominate; blurred boundary between testing and market	Close and individualized observation of patients; physicians are the principal authority ("Wer heilt hat Recht")

on legislative and regulatory controls on pharmaceuticals, during the clinical testing of specific drugs, and in the postmarket surveillance of approved medicines (Table 1). The concept of therapeutic cultures allows us to better understand the significance of networks for medical governance formed among physicians, patients, the state, and industry during the production, testing, and marketing of pharmaceutical drugs. Political interactions in the clinic that are often later "naturalized" and made invisible play an important part in the identities and social roles occupied by each of these groups.

The therapeutic cultures of the United States and Germany form the backbone of this study, and the rest of the chapters are organized around sites where they are active: legal and regulatory structures (Chapter 2), experimental methods and testing approaches (Chapters 3 and 4), and surveillance and postmarket controls (Chapter 5). Each of these areas is presented chronologically, thereby offering three different passes through the same historical period. The conclusion explores how findings from each of these arenas relate to contemporary plans for international regulatory harmonization, and speak to the future of relations among the state, physicians, industry, and patients.

Regulations governing drug approvals were instituted under different political conditions and promote distinctive methods for testing drugs in the United States and Germany. Chapter 2 describes the passage and implementation of laws regulating pharmaceuticals in the two countries. In the United States, a political construction of patients as "guinea pigs" in the wake of highly visible medical tragedies led to the rapid approval of laws that strengthened the FDA's authority over both industry and the medical profession. After the agency implemented a strict division between test and market, patient activists protested slow drug approvals and brought about important policy changes. Ger-

TABLE 2 / CASE STUDIES—MARKET AUTHORIZATION

Case Study	United States	Germany
Case 1. Terramycin	1950	1951
Case 2. Thalidomide	Not approved by the FDA in 1960s 1998—moderate to severe erythema nodosum leprosum (ENL) in leprosy	1957
Case 3. Propranolol	1967—arrhythmia 1974—angina pectoris and hypertension	1965
Case 4. Interleukin-2	1992—metastatic renal cell carcinoma 1997—metastatic melanoma	1989
Case 5. Indinavir	1996	1996

man drug laws, in contrast, were linked to broader concerns in the health care system regarding the distribution of authority across the network of physicians, industry, and the state. Since physicians had more control over constructions of "the patient," few groups articulated political demands for either greater regulatory protections or speedier drug approvals.

From the macropolitics of legislation and regulation, we shift to the narrower domain of clinical trials. Case studies of Terramycin, thalidomide, and propranolol in Chapter 3 reveal that clinical trials served different functions in the therapeutic cultures of the United States and Germany (Table 2). The FDA enforced the use of quantitative testing methods and imposed methods for statistical evaluation of test results between 1950 and 1980. Formal testing procedures were a means to demonstrate objectivity and helped shield the agency from criticism and public controversy. In Germany, on the other hand, trials were integral to defining physicians' authority in relation to the state and key to establishing new professional norms for medical care after World War II. Clinical trials carried out in the period between 1950 and the mid-1970s were generally integrated into overall patient care in Germany, rather than forming distinctive testing sites as in the United States.

Chapter 4 describes how clinical trials underwent important changes in both countries between 1980 and 2000, as evidenced by the case studies of interleukin-2 and indinavir. The emergence of patient activists and disease-based interest groups in the United States led to a new politics of testing and care. Meticulously designed clinical trials that excluded large domains of patients' lived experiences were challenged as irrelevant to "real world" drug use.

Methods used to generate knowledge about a given drug's actions in humans consequently changed to reflect arguments posed by patients, activists, and disease-based interest groups. In Germany, there were fewer changes of this kind. Instead, governance of the clinical setting by the medical profession remained comparatively intact throughout this period. No disease-based activists challenged tested methods, and medical elites continued to determine safety and efficacy in much the same way as in earlier eras. Even the establishment of a pan-European regulatory agency had little impact on the German clinical domain.

Since the mid-1950s, a growing emphasis on observing patient-drug interactions for medicines on the market has extended the boundaries of testing beyond clinical trials into routine drug therapy. Chapter 5 compares approaches to collecting, reviewing, and responding to side effects in the two countries. In the United States, the medical profession initially played an important role in this area. By the late 1960s, however, the FDA increasingly took over this task as the agency centralized and standardized mechanisms for dealing with adverse reactions. In Germany, on the other hand, the medical profession maintained a significant position in collecting and responding to adverse reaction reports, despite recent expansion of government involvement. Differences between their therapeutic cultures explain why the United States adopted a state-centered approach, while Germany vested political and regulatory authority in the medical profession.

The conclusion explores further the different ways in which American and German citizens mobilize around medical treatment and new drug approvals as points of entry for policy change. Different structures for interest group activity and different interactions in the networks that make up therapeutic cultures are particularly salient in light of current efforts to promote international regulatory harmonization. The complex interrelationships that have been built up over the past fifty years among physicians, patients, industry, and government agencies in each country will not be displaced by technical standardization alone. Instead, greater accommodation of patients' perspectives must be an integral part of the policies promoted by international agreements.

2

Drug Laws and
Therapeutic Cultures

PHARMACEUTICAL REGULATION IN THE UNITED STATES
and Germany operates at a similar level by establishing a broad
requirement that drugs be safe and effective. Neither country specifies performance standards for medicines according to the diseases
they treat, for example, by requiring antibiotics to kill a certain
amount of bacteria in a given time. Nor do regulations specify desired biochemical reactions within the body, for example, by requiring anticancer agents to reduce tumors to a specified size. Even
efficacy standards do not set precise physiological outcomes. Instead, regulations in the two countries control how, where, and
under what conditions medicines will be tested. Legislative bodies,
government agencies, and the medical profession expect clinical
tests—both before and after drugs are marketed—to weed out unsafe or ineffective pharmaceuticals.

Drug laws passed in the two countries over the course of the
twentieth century set limits on the claims manufacturers can make
about their products and narrowed the range of professional experts
who could pass judgment on new medicines. They also established
when testing ends and marketing begins. These legislative mandates

display a similar ambivalence toward the pharmaceutical industry in each country. Trust in testing procedures and the recognition of the public's need for new drugs are offset by distrust of corporate motives and public fears arising from historical cases of drug-related tragedies.

These similarities, however, are overshadowed by differences in the legal frameworks and cultural styles for regulating new medicines in the United States and Germany. A review of major regulatory laws enacted in the two countries since 1900 shows contrasts in the timing and content of legislative interventions, the influence and authority of interest groups, and in constructions of "the patient" as a citizen and consumer. This chapter first tracks these three features in the United States for laws passed in 1906, 1938, and 1962, as well as in specific regulations implemented by the Food and Drug Administration (FDA) in the 1980s and 1990s. We next examine German drug laws from 1943, 1961, 1964, and 1976, along with recent changes in the balance of power among the government, the medical profession, and the pharmaceutical industry.

Regulatory laws described here are a key site for the influence of each country's therapeutic culture on pharmaceutical regulation and the practice of medicine. The U.S. Congress increased the FDA's authority and mandated formal rules for drug evaluation in response to precipitating events, notably cases of widespread adverse drug reactions. Historically, legislative interventions were predicated on the notion that patients must be protected by the state from the worst ravages of free-market capitalism. Congress and the FDA expected government control over premarket testing to protect patients otherwise open to abuses by industry and the medical profession. In recent years, however, patients represented by disease-based organizations have agitated for greater access to drugs and speedier approvals. A firm boundary between testing and marketing—established by legislative initiatives and implemented rigorously by FDA officials—then was softened to allow for greater access to new medicines.

In Germany, on the other hand, the medical profession exercised a monopoly over constructions of "the patient" and drug laws codified existing power-sharing arrangements. Instead of the state claiming authority over premarket testing, it acted as one member of a network overseeing pharmaceutical drugs. A flexible boundary between testing and market was predicated on informal trial protocols, a structured system for collecting reports of adverse reactions, and compromises among organized interests and government officials. Because the medical profession successfully maintained and even expanded its authority to speak for the patient in the post–World War II era, few activist groups or other disease-based organizations mobilized to change the regulatory system.

Differences between therapeutic cultures in the two countries shaped the political setting for crafting and implementing drug laws. Laws then divided authority and established formal means of communication among patients, physicians, drug manufacturers, and the state. As this chapter shows, variation in legislative and regulatory structures points to the different symbolic and institutional resources that link science and medicine to broader concerns of democratic representation in the two countries. Notably, the political role of patients and resources available to ill people seeking to articulate their positions varied in the two countries as a result of their therapeutic cultures. The United States and Germany thus exhibit striking contrasts in their regulatory approaches, despite similarities in the wording and content of laws mandating pharmaceutical safety and efficacy.

Regulatory Policy and Politics in the United States

Origins and Expansion of Central Authority

Drug regulation in the United States originated in nineteenth-century vaccine and drug importation controls. At the beginning of the twentieth century, a loose coalition of farmers, state agriculture departments, and government officials sought to increase federal oversight of foodstuff manufacturers. Harvey Wiley, chief chemist of the Department of Agriculture (USDA), supported these efforts in a series of articles that described outrageous corporate behavior. He also proposed several legislative initiatives to regulate food and drug quality.[1] A turning point in public opinion and congressional action was reached with the 1906 publication of Upton Sinclair's *The Jungle*, a best-selling book detailing the unsafe practices and unsanitary conditions in the meatpacking industry.[2] Additional support for legislative action came from President Theodore Roosevelt, who criticized misleading product labels and advised Congress to enact a law "to secure the health and welfare of the consuming public."[3] The combination of public concern and presidential attention prompted Congress to approve the 1906 Pure Food and Drug Law, which banned "the manufacture, sale, or transportation of adulterated or misbranded or poisonous or deleterious foods, drugs, medicine, and liquors."[4]

The 1906 law increased the USDA's ability to regulate manufacturers through the newly formed FDA.[5] Government agents seized mislabeled products and took legal action against companies selling tainted food or drugs. Even though the agency did not have the authority to require or oversee drug tests, the 1906 law codified an earlier practice whereby pharmacists and physicians at the United States Pharmacopoeia (USP) and National Formulary (NF) set standards for the strength, quality, and purity of medicines. Requirements that companies meet these professional standards induced them to hire analytical chemists, pharmacists, and other scientists. Even drug firms not investing in research and new product development had to carry out quality assurance tests on their products.[6]

During the next two decades, FDA officials found it difficult to carry out their mandate to prevent "mislabeling or misbranding," since they had neither the budget to test products in-house nor the authority to require manufacturers to provide testing results. Without a precise breakdown of contents, the agency could not even determine the accuracy of product labels. When officials interpreted the law broadly in an effort to block drugs containing ingredients the USP or NF had declared unsafe or ineffective, the Supreme Court undermined their efforts. In a pivotal case, the justices held in 1911 that the claims of a putative cancer cure were not false labeling, since the content listing was accurate. Other court decisions through the 1930s similarly held that therapeutic claims were outside the government's regulatory control.

Responding to this weakness in the legislation, a group of FDA officials, USDA lawyers, and outside consultants gathered in 1933 to draft a new bill. They proposed expanding the government's authority to inspect manufacturers and require firms to carry out safety tests before marketing their products.[7] These provisions generated vigorous opposition among a large but decentralized group of food, drug, and cosmetic companies. While these companies were generally small and not organized in a single industry association, their broad distribution across the country guaranteed that nearly every congressional representative heard from firms opposed to the bill. At the same time, the FDA and its allies in Congress had little success in mobilizing public sentiment or broader congressional support. The bill then languished in the House Commerce Committee for five years, though Senator Royal Copeland (D-N.Y.) reintroduced it in each new legislative session.

In the mid-1930s, public and congressional attention turned to drugs and cosmetics as the result of both a clever exhibit and a tragic case of tainted medicine. As a federal agency, the FDA is prohibited from spending public funds to directly lobby members of Congress. Sidestepping this prohibition, the agency set up an exhibit in the Capitol building in 1936 that displayed labels and advertisements from harmful products next to photos of injured consumers. Described by journalists as a "chamber of horrors," the exhibit drew a wide viewership.[8]

Additional public fear of unsafe medicines arose in the wake of the Sulfanilamide disaster of 1937. This drug was one of a new class of compounds— the sulfa drugs—used to treat infectious diseases beginning in the 1930s. Initially developed at the German conglomerate I. G. Farben, sulfa drugs were imported to the United States accompanied by reports of dramatic success in treating serious infections. By 1937, American firms were selling the new antibiotics in a variety of forms, including tablets, powders, and liquids.

Tragedy struck when a scientist at S. E. Massengill used diethylene glycol, a sweet-tasting but toxic chemical, to prepare the medicine in syrup form. Although chemists at the firm examined their "Elixir of Sulfanilamide" for appearance, flavor, and fragrance, they did not test larger doses on animals, or even review published literature on solvents. After over one hundred people—mostly children—died from taking the compound, public uproar prompted Congress to take a more serious look at Copeland's bill.[9] FDA officials who examined the case initially blamed Massengill but soon widened their criticism to attack testing practices across the pharmaceutical industry. They also criticized doctors for inappropriate prescribing practices, noting that Sulfanilamide's use was "especially difficult to justify . . . in such conditions as Bright's disease [inflammation of the kidneys], bichloride of mercury poisoning, renal colic, and backache."[10] The agency used publicity associated with the Sulfanilamide case to insist on government oversight of premarket safety tests. At the same time, officials sought to gain authority over the medical profession, arguing that doctors were recklessly prescribing new medicines to patients who did not need them.

Once approved by Congress, the 1938 law significantly expanded the FDA's authority over the marketing of new drugs. Officials were required to review pre-clinical and clinical test results. They could block a drug's approval by requesting additional testing data or by formally refusing to allow its marketing: "If the secretary finds . . . that the investigations . . . which are submitted . . . do not include adequate tests by all methods reasonably applicable to show whether or not such drug is safe for use under the conditions prescribed, recommended, or suggested in the proposed labeling thereof . . . he shall, prior to the effective date of the application, issue an order refusing to permit the application to become effective."[11] After 1938, pharmaceutical regulation shifted toward prevention, since manufacturers had to produce evidence of a drug's safety before it could be given to patients. Congress did not specify precisely what kinds of tests were expected for this purpose, leaving FDA officials free to determine testing protocols in collaboration with the medical profession and pharmaceutical industry. A final provision of the law granted the agency explicit authority to conduct factory inspections. Increased federal oversight of drug companies and their products thus came about through a combination of FDA efforts and public outcry following deaths from a toxic preparation masquerading as a "miracle drug."

When implementing the 1938 law, FDA officials relied heavily on an elite cadre of physicians who had sought for decades to make medicine more scientific. As described by the historian Harry Marks, "therapeutic reformers" promoted greater use of laboratory tests, animal experiments, and clinical trials in humans to produce data on new drugs.[12] They also contributed to a crusading culture at the agency. Even with the assistance of members from the AMA Council on Pharmacy and Chemistry, the FDA had difficulty establishing uniform testing methods in the 1940s and 1950s. In the eyes of FDA officials and physicians at elite university clinics, drug testing needed to be standardized through controlled clinical trials. As described in the next chapter, adherence to this methodology varied widely during and after World War II. Medical officers generally had to make approval decisions based on qualitative assessments by the sponsoring company and case reports from physicians, rather than on the basis of statistical evaluations. FDA employees worked under strict time pressure, since objections to an application had to be made within sixty days to prevent a medicine from gaining market access.

Agency officials balanced the safety and usefulness of new drugs against their potential to harm the public through inappropriate use or adverse reactions. According to Marks, "In determining a drug's safety, FDA officials would apply a utilitarian calculus: a 'safe' drug was one whose proposed use would benefit patients more than it harmed them."[13] Consequently, the FDA's safety assessments were tied to concerns about a drug's benefits, even though there was no efficacy mandate in the law. The law was oriented toward consumer protection, but in a somewhat roundabout manner. FDA officials were to ensure that companies provided truthful statements of the contents of their therapies. Practicing physicians and pharmacists then could interpret this material in light of an individual patient's therapeutic needs. In the legislative and regulatory context, "the patient" was seen as a member of an easily misled public that needed protection by the government and professional societies. To ensure that patients were protected from harm, FDA officials sought both to improve the flow of information to physicians and to introduce greater standardization to premarket tests.

Drugs in the Regulatory State

Government efforts to improve the quality of information available about new drugs were confounded by rapid expansion of the pharmaceutical market during the 1950s. Many competing broad-spectrum antibiotics were on the market within a decade of penicillin's successful introduction in the mid-1940s. Physicians and regulators often had difficulty differentiating them from one another, especially in light of exaggerated claims made by manufacturers. Pharmaceutical firms also turned to developing medicines for long-term conditions ranging from diabetes to depression. The American public gradually grew disillusioned with the pharmaceutical industry as a result of adverse reactions from widely used stimulants, tranquilizers, and other behavior-modifying medications, along with publicity concerning drug company profits and industry advertising practices.[14]

Prices were remarkably uniform among competing brands of antibiotics and other medications in the 1950s. Noting concerns about inflation across the country, the populist Democratic senator from Tennessee, Estes Kefauver, launched an investigation into a number of industry sectors starting in 1957. His primary focus was on "administered prices," a form of price-fixing by industry leaders first described by the New Deal economist Gardiner Means. Senate hearings examined consumer prices for automobiles, bread, and, starting in 1959, prescription drugs.[15]

For Kefauver, the sick individual was someone who could barely afford medicine, such as an impoverished elderly person living on Social Security who needed cortical steroids to ease pain, or a parent with sick children who needed antibiotics. Congressional action during the first half of the century had sought to protect the public from inaccurate package labels, misleading advertising, or, in extreme cases, harmful medications. Kefauver also wanted to protect "captive" consumers and "indigent" patients from companies that colluded to set high drug prices. Starting on the first day of hearings, he represented the financially stressed patient through a letter from an elderly citizen: "I could get along fairly well on my savings and social security, but the cost of medicine is so great that I can barely make ends meet. Sometimes I think I must stop taking the medicine and just die."[16] Under Kefauver's chairmanship, the hearings generated a detailed picture of research and marketing practices in the pharmaceutical industry. The primary emphasis throughout the hearings, however, remained on drug prices and immense markups between manufacturing costs and the final market price.

In fall 1961, Kefauver introduced a bill designed to foster competition among companies, increase the FDA's authority to license and inspect manufacturers, and require formal approval of drugs based on proof of their safety and effectiveness. Overriding intense opposition from the pharmaceutical industry and a number of influential senators, Kefauver also pushed for increased federal enforcement of antitrust laws and greater price competition through compulsory cross-licensing of drug patents. Refusing to modify the bill to reflect industry suggestions, he sent it in its original form to the full Judiciary Committee. Its members soon removed the antitrust and patent sections. They also weakened Kefauver's proposal for an FDA approval system. Following a debate on the Senate floor during which Kefauver refused to support the revised bill, it was sent back to the Judiciary Committee for further revisions.[17] This move appeared to signal an ignominious end to Kefauver's bill, since many of the committee members opposed any effort to regulate the industry.

At this point, reports of birth defects linked to the sedative thalidomide began appearing in American newspapers. In what would become the century's best-known and most extensively studied drug disaster, thalidomide's use by pregnant women led to the birth of approximately 10,000 children with congenital abnormalities between 1959 and 1963.[18] Defects included stunted arms and legs, and misshapen hands and feet coupled in some cases to internal organ damage. Although only seventeen cases were registered in the United States, attention to the drug breathed new life into Kefauver's bill. Initial newspaper reports indicated that the 1938 U.S. law had protected the public, because FDA officials prevented domestic marketing of the drug.[19] During the summer of 1962, however, a scandal emerged concerning both the widespread distribution of thalidomide to physicians as an "experimental" drug and pressure brought to bear by company officials during the FDA review.

The U.S.-based pharmaceutical company William S. Merrell, Inc., licensed thalidomide from its German manufacturer, Chemie Grünenthal, in 1958. After carrying out laboratory, animal, and initial human tests, the company submitted an application to the FDA for marketing authorization. Frances Kelsey, the medical officer assigned to review the application, found deficiencies in the animal studies and criticized the company's testing methods.[20] She then requested additional toxicity tests, putting the application on hold.

During the next eleven months, Kelsey repeatedly stalled the thalidomide application by demanding that the company conduct additional long-term safety tests. Throughout this period, Merrell aggressively promoted the drug's safety with regulators and managers in the Bureau of Medicine. According to Kelsey, "Merrell contacted FDA's Bureau of Medicine fifty times in an effort to get this drug on the American market and a number of the efforts to get the New Drug Application approved were very vigorous."[21]

At one point, company officials contacted Kelsey's supervisor in an attempt to speed the approval. Two days later, they contacted Kelsey directly, "and tried to get me to say I'd agree to pass it in a day."[22] A week later, Kelsey wrote the firm that she had read reports from Europe describing cases of nerve damage among patients using thalidomide. When Kelsey accused the company of intentionally withholding this information, Merrell's representative threatened to sue the agency, calling her statement "libelous." Kelsey nonetheless held her ground and repeatedly demanded additional data until the company eventually withdrew its application in March 1962.

In an effort to meet Kelsey's requests, but also as part of a plan to woo physicians, Merrell distributed over two million thalidomide tablets to some 1,200 practicing doctors. Ostensibly part of its investigation into the drug's safety and efficacy, Merrell's broad distribution looked to FDA officials like a marketing program, not a clinical study. Merrell's unsupervised investigational study came under sharp criticism when journalists and FDA officials questioned its ethical assumptions. For example, in a series of widely read *Saturday Review* articles, John Lear portrayed patients as exploited "guinea pigs" and demanded greater government oversight of the testing process: "They [pharmaceutical firms] pick the experimenters, decide the number of same, and are free to accept or reject anyone's claim to qualifications and facilities. They may begin using drugs on humans before safety has been established through animal tests, and they have the privilege of keeping the patients in ignorance throughout, lest knowledge of the guinea pig status have some undesirable psychological effect on the results of the experiment."[23]

Public attitudes toward consumer protection and legislative definitions of the patient both underwent significant changes as details emerged regarding the close call with thalidomide. From concern with the ability of elderly Americans to pay for medicines, attention shifted to premarket testing, protections for research subjects, and the ability of FDA officials to shield the public from dangerous drugs. Whereas Kefauver sought to help consumers by forcing intellectual property exchanges among drug firms, Lear and others called for protection of patients from physicians and companies alike. Reports of the magnitude of the tragedy in Europe soon aligned support behind an increase in the FDA's regulatory authority over drug testing.

Drug testing provisions from Kefauver's bill then were combined with consumer protection legislation advocated by President John Kennedy and introduced as a separate bill by Representative Oren Harris (D-Ark.). Following unanimous approval in both the House and Senate, Kennedy signed the Kefauver-Harris Amendments to the Food and Drug Act into law in October 1962 (Figure 1). The FDA now was authorized to set standards for every stage of new drug testing, from the laboratory to human trials. In an important departure from the past, government officials had to approve a new drug—or make an exception for clinical testing—before any patient could take it.

In order to shore up its scientific and medical legitimacy for this expanded regulatory role, the agency greatly increased its use of advisory committees. Experts with solid research credentials were chosen from outside the FDA to review specific new drug applications as well as general procedures for testing and decision making at the agency. As Sheila Jasanoff has noted, advisory committees helped shield the agency from the criticism that its regulatory decisions lacked scientific merit: "The formidable array of expert advisory committees associated with the agency since the late 1960s testifies to its recognition that legitimation from the independent scientific community is indispensable to the success of its regulatory programs."[24]

FDA officials expected that committee members would also "convey to their professional colleagues facts concerning the intent and methods of achiev-

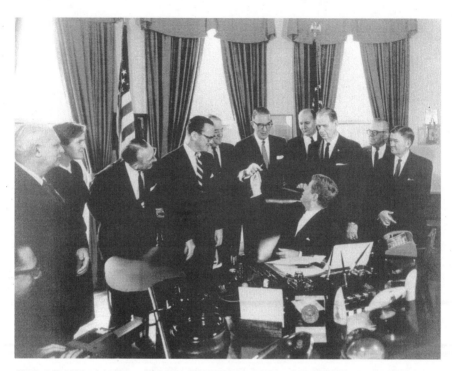

Figure 1. President John Kennedy signing the 1962 Kefauver-Harris Amendments to the Food and Drug Act into law. He is handing the pen to Estes Kefauver; Frances Kelsey is second from the left. (FDA History Office)

ing the improved control of investigational drugs."[25] Advisory committees thus were intended to work as two-way streets: advice should flow to the FDA from professionals, but these experts should also publicize and promote FDA-mandated methods for clinical testing broadly across the medical community.

Unlike the 1938 statute, the 1962 law explicitly stated that the FDA should rely on scientific testing of new drugs.[26] Once the FDA began enforcing these provisions, pharmaceutical companies had to change their pre-clinical testing practices, establish formal agreements with physicians to carry out clinical trials, and employ complex statistical evaluations to demonstrate drug safety and efficacy. Clinical investigations by law involved three phases: first, dosage tests in a small number of healthy subjects, second, initial trials on a limited number of patients, and third, two or more controlled clinical trials.[27] Physicians directing drug trials also had to follow government guidelines for "good clinical practices." The FDA thus took on responsibilities for setting testing standards previously exercised by professional bodies such as the AMA Council on Drugs, the U.S. Pharmacopoeia, and the National Formulary. Physicians carrying out clinical trials or advising the agency increasingly were engaged as individual "experts," rather than as members of a professional collective.

As gatekeepers, FDA officials had the authority to postpone or deny new drug applications. Responding to fear of the next thalidomide-like disaster, this feature of the 1962 law promoted a precautionary model of regulatory review. Premarket testing emerged as a controlled domain for producing knowledge about drug safety and efficacy, increasing the amount of time between the invention and marketing of new medicines. Within a decade, critics claimed that FDA regulations were harming innovation at drug companies and weakening industrial competitiveness. Studies carried out by the economists Samuel Peltzman and Henry Grabowski in the early 1970s, for example, found a striking decline in the number of new drugs invented and approved for human use after the mid-1960s. They concluded that research opportunities were drying up and, more significantly, that government regulation had produced a precipitous drop in innovation at American pharmaceutical firms.[28] Free-market economist Milton Friedman estimated the costs of drug regulation to consumers at $250 million per year: "It is as if a 5 to 10 percent tax were levied on drug sales and the money so raised were spent on invisible monuments to the late Senator Kefauver."[29]

Physicians became concerned that new medicines were reaching European patients earlier than Americans; indeed, two prominent doctors, William Wardell and Louis Lasagna, found delays in the regulatory approval of new drugs in the United States compared to European countries. Wardell coined the term "drug lag" to characterize this delay, arguing that patients in France, Germany, and the United Kingdom could get new drugs up to two years before Americans.[30] Differences in drug approval times, Wardell and Lasagna argued, indicated that American patients were missing out on useful medicines, especially for treating cardiovascular, diuretic, respiratory, and gastro-intestinal ailments. These critics described regulatory impacts in terms of public suffering and even attributed several thousand deaths to delays in the approval of beta-blockers such as propranolol and practolol.[31] In contrast to economists' focus on risks to innovation and the competitive standing of American pharmaceutical companies, physicians described sick patients as facing the most salient risks from overregulation.

Claims regarding public health and patients' access to drugs attracted congressional attention, and both Wardell and Lasagna were cited frequently in proposals to reform the FDA. Responding to critics, FDA authorities argued that subjecting large numbers of people to drugs of unknown danger would harm more patients than slow approvals.[32] The primary policy lesson FDA officials drew from the thalidomide case was to emphasize premarket testing and avoid approving drugs with side effects. Officials at the agency only rarely faced public criticism or congressional inquiry for denying specific medicines to ill people. As Commissioner Alexander Schmidt explained in 1974, "In all our history, we are unable to find one instance where a Congressional hearing investigated the failure of FDA to approve a new drug."[33] In contrast, dozens of hearings in the House and Senate during the 1960s and 1970s sought to expose the dangers posed by unsafe or ineffective drugs, and congressional leaders regularly advised the agency to exercise greater caution before approving medicines.[34]

The drug lag debate did make visible a dilemma faced by American regulators in deciding between long premarket review and potentially widespread adverse reactions. Although the agency tilted heavily toward precaution during the 1970s and early 1980s, debates about regulatory trade-offs contributed to an atmosphere in which a vocal group of patients and activists could produce significant changes.

Bringing the Patient Back In

Unlike earlier cases of improper drug testing or unauthorized use of people as research subjects, patients with rare diseases, breast cancer, and AIDS began to speak out for themselves in the 1980s. The National Organization for Rare Disorders spearheaded a drive for the 1983 Orphan Drug Act, which gave pharmaceutical companies increased commercial exclusivity, tax credits for research, and direct financial aid for clinical trials of medicines to treat diseases affecting fewer than 200,000 people nationwide.[35] Likewise, patients began forging national organizations that compiled data on disease rates, lobbied for greater research funding, and agitated for policy change. For example, the National Breast Cancer Coalition held frequent fund-raising campaigns to support research, called on Congress to increase the budget of the National Institutes of Health, and demanded regulatory changes to increase the availability of new treatments.[36]

HIV-AIDS ultimately provoked an even more visible crisis in American drug regulation, pitting activists and patients against an agency supposedly acting in their interests. Groups including the New York Gay Men's Health Crisis, San Francisco's Project Inform, and chapters of the AIDS Coalition to Unleash Power (ACT UP) protested slow drug approval rates and urged faster infusion of "drugs into bodies."[37] Larry Kramer, the well-known author and activist, famously linked drug approval to patient survival: "There is no question on the part of anyone fighting AIDS that the FDA consists of the single most incomprehensible bottleneck in American bureaucratic history—one that is actually prolonging the roll call of death."[38] Activists drew upon a coherent

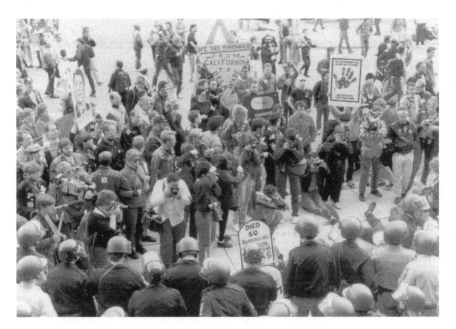

Figure 2. FDA protest, 1988. (FDA History Office)

group identity among gay men forged over decades of opposition to the American cultural and political mainstream. They also enrolled scientists and physicians familiar with drug regulation to support their cause.

In a rare public demonstration against a consumer protection agency, a large rally was held at FDA headquarters in October 1988 (Figure 2). The protest prompted greater government recognition of the seriousness and legitimacy of activists' demands for more rapid drug approvals. ACT UP's Treatment and Data Committee informed fellow activists about the agency and provided detailed explanations of their demands to television and radio programs. Activists prepared provocative visual aids, and photographs of protesters lying in front of FDA headquarters drew national attention. In the words of one activist, "government agencies dealing with AIDS, particularly the FDA and NIH, began to listen to us, to include us in decision-making, even to ask for our input."[39] The "professionalization of treatment activism" that resulted from this dialogue with the FDA and NIH ultimately led many AIDS patients to marginalize alternative therapies and instead focus their attention on reforming the mainstream pharmaceutical industry and government regulations.

By the time of the protest at its headquarters, the FDA had already begun to change the drug approval process in an effort to shorten review times. The primary anti-AIDS drug AZT (Zidovudine) was distributed to more than 4,000 patients in 1986 and gained marketing approval after just 107 days of FDA review; this was reported widely as the fastest approval on record for a major therapeutic product.[40] A year later, the agency issued the first in a series of rules intended to expedite the availability of experimental drugs, known as treatment investigational new drug (treatment IND) regulations. Under these provisions, companies could distribute unapproved medicines to patients with life-threatening diseases, so long as there was a "reasonable basis" for concluding that the drug was effective and would not expose patients in clinical trials to "significant additional risks."[41]

Expansion of the treatment IND regulations in 1988 and 1990 made experimental drugs more accessible to AIDS patients, including those not participating in clinical trials.[42] Soon thereafter, the FDA formally adopted a system for "parallel track" review, allowing officials to approve drugs prior to the final review of safety and efficacy data.[43] Parallel track initially provided drugs to AIDS patients who were not taking part in clinical trials. It was later broadened to allow private physicians to prescribe medicines to HIV-positive individuals not yet exhibiting symptoms of full-blown AIDS. An "accelerated approval" plan announced at the end of 1992 gave even greater leeway for officials to approve drugs based on surrogate endpoints rather than traditional measures of safety and efficacy.[44]

The Patient in Regulatory and Legislative Settings

Three major shifts occurred in the status of "the patient" during the twentieth century. Each of these shaped drug regulation and redefined the authority of physicians, industry, and the state (Table 3). First, in the wake of the Sulfanilamide tragedy, patients were seen as needing state and professional protection from unethical drug manufacturers through improved information. The 1938 statute therefore outlawed the mislabeling of drugs and provided medical professionals with accurate information on the contents of a medical preparation. In the second shift, following the near miss with thalidomide, patients were viewed as needing protection from industry and from easily duped physicians through direct government intervention. The 1962 law thus required greater FDA control over every aspect of drug discovery and testing.

More recently, activist groups and disease-based organizations have presented patients as sophisticated "rational actors" who can review medical information and make informed decisions for themselves. Changes in FDA regulations consequently shifted certain aspects of risk evaluation and decision-making control to patients and physicians. Initiatives since the peak of political attention to the AIDS crisis in the early 1990s, notably the 1992 Prescription Drug User Fee Act (PDUFA) and the 1997 FDA Modernization Act (FDAMA),

TABLE 3 / TURNING POINTS IN AMERICAN DRUG REGULATION

Year	Law/Regulation	Primary Focus and Key Provisions
1906	Pure Food and Drug Law	Adulteration and misbranding of food and drugs: a) FDA reviews food and drug labels b) FDA can seize or withdraw improperly labeled products from the market
1938	Federal Food, Drug, and Cosmetic Act	Drug safety: a) Manufacturers must conduct tests to prove a drug is safe b) FDA has 60 days to review applications and file objections or pose questions, otherwise new drug is considered approved
1962	Kefauver-Harris Amendments	Drug efficacy and safety: a) FDA must approve a drug prior to marketing b) FDA can require market withdrawals c) FDA sets standards for every stage of drug testing from laboratory to clinic d) FDA defines "Good Manufacturing Practice" and is required to inspect plants
1988 **1990**	Treatment Investigational New Drug Regulations Parallel Track Review	Relaxing the boundary between test and market: a) Companies can give unapproved medicines to patients with life-threatening diseases b) FDA can approve a new drug prior to final compilation of safety and efficacy data

have promoted rapid drug approvals at the agency.[45] PDUFA authorized "user fees," whereby the FDA charges companies to review applications in exchange for tighter adherence to deadlines. The FDAMA included measures intended to reduce clinical study time and "fast track authority" to quickly process applications for priority drugs.[46] These acts also support a consumerist vision for the patient by requiring drug companies and the FDA to produce and distribute information helpful to patients who want to make individual decisions about disease treatment.

The expansion of direct-to-consumer advertisements during the past five years has only served to reinforce this trend of putting patients into the role of "informed purchasers" of health care products.[47] Critics argue that this can run counter to patients' best interests. For example, physicians have noted a rapid increase in requests for specific drugs, including cases where patients ask for completely inappropriate treatments.[48] A recent report to the pharmaceutical industry on ways to improve direct advertising thus recommends depth of content, accuracy, and objectivity as key to "personalized health solutions and support." These, in turn, will "increase the likelihood of patients requesting products and driving sales growth."[49] This American construction of "the patient" contrasts sharply with developments in Germany and Europe.

German Regulatory Governance

Drug regulation in Germany typically occasions fewer conflicts among industry, the medical profession, and the government than have been common in the United States. Historically, associations representing physicians and pharmacists served as intermediaries between patients and the state. They also mediated between the pharmaceutical industry and government health officials and played a major role in deciding which drugs were on the market. Strikingly, this system tended to hide "the patient" from legislative debates on new drug laws. Physicians were rarely challenged when they argued for public protection by means of professional standards and self-regulation within the medical community.

Over the course of the twentieth century, a succession of governments nevertheless gradually centralized key aspects of drug review and registration. In contrast to the United States, however, government officials did not offer alternative constructions of patients in order to expand their control over drug testing. The distribution of authority and responsibility across a network of industry, the medical profession, and the state made it difficult for patients themselves to articulate their positions in new ways. In recent years, individual critics have raised issues similar to those articulated by disease activists in the United States, but few organizations formed in Germany to force changes in the regulatory system.

Local versus Central Control

During the Second Empire (1871–1918) and under the Weimar Republic (1919–33), national drug regulations were limited to manufacturing and distribution controls that established boundaries between pharmacists and physicians. An 1872 act defined pharmaceuticals as "substances for the treatment of illness in humans or animals," and restricted their sale to recognized apothecaries.[50] Laws instituted by individual states and the national government prior to the 1940s did not require manufacturers to list ingredients on drug labels or restrict advertising claims. Instead, the government controlled public access to pharmaceuticals by establishing who could prescribe and sell drugs. Five proposals for greater government oversight of drug manufacturing and advertising all failed between 1928 and 1941, primarily because of industry opposition.[51]

Cozy relations between the pharmaceutical industry and the government changed radically in February 1943, when the Nazi government banned all new drugs, aside from medicines granted special approval by the Ministry of Defense. This Stop-Verordnung centralized government control over the pharmaceutical market in one fell swoop:

§1. Effective immediately, the manufacture of new pharmaceutical products (specialties) is banned.

§2. As defined by this decree, pharmaceutical products (specialties) are substances and preparations intended for the prevention, mitigation, or cure of diseases, suffering, bodily harm, or complaints among persons or animals that are marketed in packaged form and with special designs, or are marketed as trade-name goods by manufacturers.[52]

In effect, the national government claimed authority over drug research, testing, and marketing. Three months later, a revision to the Stop-Verordnung more narrowly specified which medicines its provisions covered. The government banned research or production of anesthetics, analgesics for use in pregnancy or among the elderly, diagnostic devices, and disinfectants.[53]

The timing of these two decrees coincided with an overall shift in the Nazi government and German economy to a condition of "total war." A looming catastrophe for the German army in the east and the launch of allied air raids from the north and west put significant pressure on Hitler's war economy by early 1943. At the same time, the Nazi leadership was concerned about public opinion and support for war efforts at home. Joseph Goebbels then changed the government's propaganda strategy from reassuring the populace that all was well to confronting Germans with the possibility of defeat. He offered the public an alternative of total victory or utter destruction in his famous *Sportpalast* speech, given just one week after the Stop-Verordnung was issued.[54] The home front was thus primed to make sacrifices for the war effort.

Prohibiting the development of medicines to ease suffering or heal the ill served a number of intertwined purposes for the Nazi regime. First, denying care was an additional step in the eugenicist program of weeding out "sick" and "degenerate" members from the idealized Aryan race.[55] Second, preventing companies from expending research and development efforts on "useless or even harmful pharmaceuticals" freed additional raw materials and personnel for wartime production.[56] Third, Nazi administrators felt that the experience of physical pain would remind citizens of suffering at the front. Goebbels and other officials responsible for morale felt that this would help solidify opinion behind the military. By 1943, the German patient had been reconceived, in effect, as a body that should experience the pain and suffering of war.

Though the first decree had banned the introduction of all new medicines, the revised version provided for a formal "exception permit." Under this arrangement, manufacturers could apply to the Interior Ministry for an official license to produce a new drug. Applications had to include information on the labeling, composition, form, packaging, dosage, and intended use of the medicine along with documentation of its pharmacological and clinical efficacy. These features provided the first national controls over drug testing and manufacturing in Germany. At the same time, they limited the role of physicians in making determinations of drug safety or efficacy. Authority was instead centralized in the hands of Nazi bureaucrats.

In the decade following World War II, West Germany underwent a remarkably rapid transition from the dictatorial Nazi government to a thriving democracy. Not surprisingly, state control of industry, professions, and civil society was largely discredited. Ministries of the newly founded Federal Republic were cautious in asserting their authority. In industrial sectors ranging from steel and coal to pharmaceuticals, emergent labor unions and reorganized professional associations filled the void created by the receding state.[57] The market economy that arose during the economic boom of the *Wirtschaftswunder* therefore was tempered by a social welfare state with weak regulatory controls coupled to strong professional associations and labor unions.

A tripartite division of power emerged among industry, the Interior Ministry, and the Federal Chamber of Physicians (Bundesärztekammer, or BÄK) in the pharmaceutical sector. Ministry officials initially sought to maintain the Stop-Verordnung as a basis for controlling pharmaceutical companies. Frustrated by this sweeping ban on new products, industry representatives took the unusual step of arguing in favor of a new drug law. Recognizing that a procedure for registering new drugs with a central authority would be preferable to a ban on research and production, the industry turned to pre-war debates over a drug law. In a letter to the Interior Ministry, its trade association argued: "The decree cannot be seen as a substitute for the registration procedure that the pharmaceutical law, which could not be enacted due to wartime conditions, had foreseen."[58] Since the medical profession and industry each saw opportunities to expand its authority, consensus on a new drug law proved elusive during the 1950s. Proposals for legislation did not even enter discussion in the German parliament (Bundestag).

At the same time, industry representatives challenged the Stop-Verordnung in court and brought political pressure to bear in support of either an unregulated free-market system or a low-key registration procedure. Their efforts were largely unsuccessful. Interior ministers argued convincingly that the older statute provided necessary controls over the industry's tendency to market unnecessary or dangerous medicines: "The decree from 11. February 1943 may well be based on wartime raw material scarcity. It nevertheless, above all, has health policy purposes to fulfill. Control can be achieved over new pharmaceutical products in order to protect the populace from too many choices and injury. This provision of the decree . . . is as vital today as in 1943."[59]

Carrying the ban on new drugs into the 1950s, however, did not mean that no new medicines were available to German patients. Manufacturers readily obtained permission to market new drugs from the newly organized Federal Health Office (Bundesgesundheitsamt, or BGA), including antibiotics licensed from U.S. firms.[60] Keeping the law on the books provided the new German government with a means to oversee pharmaceutical companies and claim an interest in protecting consumers. At the same time, the fledgling Federal Republic did little to enforce the Stop-Verordnung's provisions.

The risks of patients becoming ill or dying from poorly tested medicines were comparatively unimportant to German regulatory politics during this period. Sulfa drugs used in the 1930s were accompanied by many adverse reactions, but this was seen only as further evidence of the need for professional autonomy. Physicians could even argue that regulation by means of professional associations succeeded in preventing events analogous to the Sulfanilamide disaster in the United States. The Nazi Stop-Verordnung drastically changed the balance of regulatory authority for only a few years. Physicians and industry officials soon reasserted much of their authority. Dismissing government oversight, they argued that safe drug therapy relied on expert care and consideration of the individual case by a professional. No interest groups arose to advance the cause of "suffering patients" or "inadequately informed consumers." Instead, economic concerns and the balance of power among the state, medical community, and pharmaceutical industry dominated debates over regulatory policy.

Networked Drug Regulation

Federal regulations or, more specifically, the absence of government control of the pharmaceutical industry took center stage in the early 1960s. The Federal Constitutional Court nullified the Stop-Verordnung in 1959, not because of its connection to the Nazi government but rather due to the excessive "authority and discretion" it concentrated in a single government ministry.[61] According to the high court, the lack of formal criteria for granting exceptions to the Stop-Verordnung precluded impartial decision making at the BGA. In the absence of a federal statute, the West German states individually established registration laws for new pharmaceuticals.

Seeking to rationalize the ensuing patchwork of regulations, both the governing Christian-Democratic Union (CDU) and opposition Social-Democratic Party (SPD) proposed federal drug laws in 1958.[62] A parliamentary advisory committee redrafted them as a single bill in early 1959, and hearings were held in the main Health Committee. The modified bill was submitted to the full Bundestag at the end of 1960. Throughout this period, extra-parliamentary negotiations took place among ruling party members, industry representatives, and members of the BÄK. Each group brought its own concerns to the table and presented an alternative vision for German drug regulation. The industry was primarily worried about trade disadvantages resulting from the lack of coordination among the states. BÄK expressed concern about health risks from inadequate supervision of new drug development. At the same time, both industry and physicians regarded federal oversight as a challenge to their own authority.

Proposals for prescription drug requirements and controls over advertising claims dominated parliamentary debates. The pharmaceutical industry opposed BÄK's suggestion that all drugs with "new active substances" require a physician's prescription during an initial three-year period. Industry representatives also wanted to weaken or eliminate proposed restrictions on drug advertising. In order to get its support for the legislation, these provisions were dropped. A majority of parliamentary representatives nevertheless announced that they would support future legislation to reduce over-the-counter drug availability and regulate pharmaceutical advertising.

Under the final provisions of the 1961 Drug Law, pharmaceutical companies had to obtain a manufacturing license and register new drugs with the BGA in West Berlin. In order to do so, companies had to submit reports summarizing pharmacological and clinical tests. They also had to describe side effects associated with a new treatment. The law did not mandate specific tests, nor did it specify who should carry out drug trials. In effect, clinical trials and post-marketing review were seen as procedures best left to medical experts coordinated by the BÄK. In order to help the BGA evaluate the quality of clinical data, firms were expected to provide the names of physicians who had carried out the tests.

Sections of the 1961 law that forbade manufacturers from distributing "dangerous" medicines gave the BGA important controls over the drug market. However, it was left to industry and the medical profession to expose dangerous drugs and establish which methods were appropriate to determine safety. Furthermore, the BGA lacked any mechanism to slow or prevent a medicine from reaching the market. Instead, the government was placed in a reactive posture whereby officials could only advise companies to voluntarily withdraw drugs that proved dangerous once they were widely available.

Weaknesses in the new law became apparent within a few months when connections were drawn between thalidomide (marketed in Germany as Contergan) and an epidemic of birth defects across the country. Widespread use of the sedative, generally available without a prescription, resulted in some 4,000 cases of birth defects among German children. Publicity about Contergan's impact produced strident debates regarding the 1961 law in the Bundestag and across the country.[63] Industry, the medical profession, and the health ministry adopted very different positions on how to prevent future catastrophes. Physicians and industry representatives agreed that the responsibility for producing safe and efficacious drugs should remain with manufacturers. Nevertheless, proposals for the federal government to centralize the testing of new drugs were widely discredited as too costly, inefficient, and unlikely to guarantee product safety. Instead, organizations such as the BÄK and the German Pharmacology Society reacted to the tragedy by lobbying for greater control over drug testing.[64]

The Bundestag responded to these initiatives in 1964 with revisions that required additional premarket testing and prescription-only status for new drugs.[65] Despite a proposal advanced by the SPD to increase government oversight of drug prescriptions, the final law allowed doctors to decide individually on the best treatments for their patients. Their authority to collect and standardize reports of adverse reactions—coordinated by BÄK's Drug Commission—was also left intact. Reports from pharmacological and clinical tests had to accompany new drug registrations. Yet the BGA could not refuse a registration until the manufacturer had ample opportunity to produce convincing results. Unlike in the United States, German government officials did not use the law to require standardized tests and controlled clinical trials. BGA officials instead waited for the BÄK's Drug Commission and the German Society for Internal Medicine to issue guidelines for drug testing.[66] As part of the registration process, manufacturers had to verify that they followed these standards.

In this manner, both the 1961 and 1964 laws codified social, economic, and regulatory roles for industry, the medical profession, and the government. Companies were to produce new drugs, sponsor tests, and submit reports to the government. Physicians working at elite university clinics and in large hospitals used guidelines developed by their professional associations to carry out pharmacological and clinical tests. The BGA reviewed final reports and officials discussed test results with physicians and the company. Medicines then were registered and could be prescribed to patients around the country. This complex web of relations precluded the drawing of sharp boundaries between the state and industry, or between the state and the medical profession. Without avenues of political access, no "external" critics could demand a radical change in drug regulation, even in the wake of the public scandal associated with Contergan. Rather than increasing government-based regulatory oversight, reaction to the tragedy prompted professional groups to expand their authority over members' activities and to gradually formalize relationships with one another and the state.

Beyond Semisovereignty

Despite the apparent efficacy of this non-governmental system for oversight of pharmaceutical testing and marketing, some members of parliament were dissatisfied with the relatively weak BGA. Delegates to a 1971 SPD conference on "health politics" proposed major changes in the drug law, especially for government controls over drug testing. They charged the BGA with a pro-industry bias and demanded the formation of a "neutral" body to provide physicians with information on pharmaceutical prices and comparisons of drug efficacy.[67] Social Democrats, now in power, considered new regulations a means to address public concerns about drug safety. To gain industry support, they argued that a stronger law would increase sales by reducing public fears of side effects.

Additional motivation for the parliament to expand the drug law came from a 1965 European Commission directive to establish formal approval procedures in a national regulatory agency.[68] Although many European countries initially failed to comply with the directive, in part because it mandated approval procedures without specifying pre-clinical or clinical testing criteria, most had fallen into line by the mid-1970s. A bill to formalize safety and efficacy testing, establish price transparency, and monitor approved drugs was presented to the Bundestag in May 1974 and soon gained the ruling coalition's approval. At that point, the bill was sent to the BÄK and the pharmaceutical industry association for analysis and commentary.

The BÄK and other medical groups responded in support of increased safety and efficacy testing. Pharmaceutical companies, however, remained opposed to the government setting testing standards and objected to requirements for price comparisons among analogous medicines.[69] Once these provisions were dropped, the industry gave quiet approval to the legislation, while voicing concerns about the "bureaucratization" of drug review.[70]

Trade associations representing homeopathic and other alternative therapies, on the other hand, fought a lengthy battle to protect their interests. The proposed bill required identical tests for safety and efficacy for all medicines before review by a central regulatory authority. Arguing that their therapies could not be evaluated using "purely scientific" criteria, companies selling alternative therapies vigorously opposed the proposed legislation. Based on widely circulated petitions, publicity through posters, bumper stickers, and published opinion pieces, supporters of "therapeutic freedom" succeeded in

TABLE 4 / TURNING POINTS IN GERMAN DRUG REGULATION

Year	Law/Regulation	Primary Focus and Key Provisions
1943	Stop-Verordnung	a) Ban on the production of pharmaceuticals for all but life-threatening conditions b) Halted research into new compounds
1961	Arzneimittelgesetz I	a) Manufacturers must be licensed by the government b) New drugs must be registered with the BGA
1964	Arzneimittelgesetz II	a) Required premarket tests (overseen by clinical pharmacologists) b) Drugs with novel ingredients only available by prescription
1976	Arzneimittelgesetz III	a) BGA must approve drugs, based on quality, safety, and efficacy tests b) Medical profession sets testing standards c) Pharmaceutical companies must document the informed consent of patients participating in clinical trials and purchase special liability insurance

exempting homeopathic and natural remedies (*Naturheilmittel*) from the efficacy requirement.[71]

After revising the bill to meet these objections, the Bundestag approved it in May 1976. Even though it gained approval of the upper house within several months, the new law did not take effect until January 1978. The two-year transition period was designed to give companies and physicians time to develop and implement new methods for drug testing, especially for data collection and evaluation. In its final form, the law increased government oversight of the quality, safety, and efficacy of new drugs prior to marketing. It included separate procedures for registering homeopathic and other alternative medicines. Responsibility for setting testing standards, however, again was assigned to the medical profession. Reflecting tensions apparent since the thalidomide disaster, the law required proof of patients' informed consent prior to joining clinical trials, and forced companies to purchase special liability insurance before launching tests on humans.

Compared to earlier laws, the new Arzneimittelgesetz mandated specific testing regimens and required details about premarket tests (Table 4). Applications to the BGA had to include basic data on a drug's composition, side effects, interaction with other products, and analytical, pharmacological-toxicological, and clinical results that documented its safety and efficacy.[72] Only qualified experts—defined in the law as physicians with two or more years of clinical testing experience—could carry out trials. Physicians also had to provide an expert assessment describing "whether the drug is suitably effective in the given fields of application, whether it is tolerated, whether the prescribed dosage is proper, and which contraindications and side effects exist."[73]

Questions about the safety and efficacy of a drug thereby became insepar-able from debates about clinical trials, just as in the United States. Unlike in America, however, the criterion that tests follow "knowledge and methods cur-rently available to medical science" was used less to mandate government con-trol over a rigid methodology of double-blind, clinically controlled trials than to grant official recognition to the professional authority of the BÄK. The law included measures intended to protect patients from unsafe drugs; however, in practice officials at the BGA sought to balance risk reductions from thoroughly tested drugs against the potential for decreased new drug innovation.

In any case, since companies were not required to submit testing protocols for regulatory review, government officials could do little to mandate specific changes to premarket tests. BGA officials instead retrospectively evaluated applications to see whether the potential public benefits of a new drug out-weighed risks to individual trial subjects. Nevertheless, the office was not powerless to request additional testing, and in some cases, it flatly rejected new drug applications.[74]

Just as the FDA increased its use of advisory committees following the 1962 law, so the BGA formed "authorization commissions" to help review drug applications after 1978. Under the German law, commission members served as experts on specific topics and could make suggestions on the entire review process. The authorization commissions brought together medical experts and company representatives in regular meetings and coordinated ongoing corre-spondence among members. BGA officials could bypass commission recom-mendations. In such instances, however, they had to justify their decision to the company based on medical criteria.

Building a Therapeutic Culture

Even though the 1976 law placed premarket testing under BGA oversight, the agency was under considerable pressure from industry and the medical profession to accept their drug evaluations. As clinical pharmacology gained additional institutional recognition and stability during the 1980s, discussions about drug approval tended to take place in "closed-door" settings. This pro-cedure minimized conflict and kept drug review times short. As in the United States, the appearance and spread of AIDS posed challenges to the German regulatory system. Despite the modest number of AIDS cases in Germany when compared to the United States (Figure 3), Germans formed several new organizations to help sick people and lobby for policy change.

The networked system of regulation among government officials, the med-

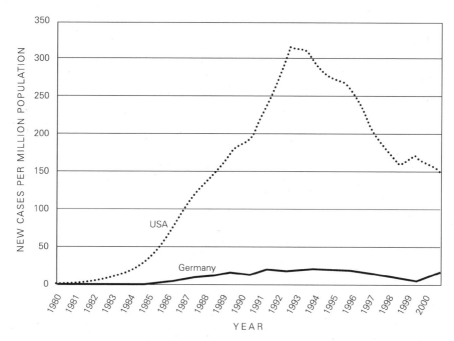

Figure 3. AIDS cases by year of reporting, 1980–2000. (Data from United Nations–World Health Organization Working Group on Global HIV/AIDS, Epidemiological Fact Sheets on HIV/AIDS and Sexually Transmitted Infections [Geneva: UNAIDS/WHO, 2002])

ical profession, and industry, however, prevented people with AIDS from easily locating a physical or administrative site for protest actions. Any apparent weakness at one node was covered by assurances by the other parties. At the same time, few symbolic resources were available with which to demand access to the regulatory process. Whereas American activists blockaded the FDA and held up gravestones marking their deaths from "FDA inertia," German AIDS patients found it difficult to articulate a stance as outsiders demanding representation in regulatory decisions.[75]

Concerned individuals—mostly gay men—mobilized volunteers in prevention and education efforts. They also provided direct assistance for patients in advanced stages of the disease. Deutsche AIDS-Hilfe, a publicly supported organization, was formed in Berlin in 1983 and soon established chapters in cities across West Germany. The group subsequently gained a monopoly position to represent AIDS patients with government officials. As a quasi-public administration, the organization rarely adopted confrontational techniques to bring about changes in public policy. Instead, as its name suggests, rather than "act up" to bring about changes to medical policy, the group sought to help patients cope with the disease.

Formation of a national AIDS advisory council, the AIDS-Beirat, likewise produced few policy changes concerning drug regulation. Supported by a federal government "eager to establish one peak body with whom they can deal," the AIDS-Beirat worked within established channels and focused its attention on public education, insurance benefits, and daily assistance for very sick AIDS patients.[76] More confrontational organizations such as ACT UP made their presence felt, but failed to attract much popular support. As the political analyst Dennis Altman points out, "Americans have been prominent in the establishment of most European ACT-UPs: it is revealing that a German book on ACT-UP . . . consisted almost entirely of pieces by Americans."[77]

Two controversies with significance for the German regulatory system nevertheless did arise in this period. First, drug manufacturers began complaining in the late 1980s of an "approval jam" (*Zulassungsstau*), comparable to the American "drug lag" critique of the early 1970s. Despite their best efforts to publicize bureaucratic inefficiency, the issue attracted little public attention beyond the Bundestag's Health Commission and the trade press. BGA officials had approved some 250 new drugs in 1987, compared to a peak of over 1,000 in 1984.[78] In an effort to shorten review times, the drug law was amended in 1989 and again in 1990. These revisions loosened testing requirements and increased the BGA's discretionary power.

Under the revised law, officials could make drugs with "significant therapeutic advances" available to patients prior to the completion of clinical testing.[79] The BGA also could ignore certain aspects of the approval process in consultation with authorization commissions. These German versions of the American "expedited approval" process were used to grant market access to AZT and other AIDS drugs. By 1992, the BGA was approving drugs more rapidly, but still had a backlog of over 8,000 applications to review. The Bundestag's Health Commission then recommended technical changes in the review process to increase computer use and ease communication among different BGA branches.[80] Notably, the issue did not move beyond a tight network of industry and government experts and was not used by AIDS groups to agitate for changes in the regulatory process.

In a second development of potential significance for German regulatory politics, failure to test the nation's blood supply allowed HIV to spread among hemophiliacs and other recipients of blood transfusions in the late 1980s. The resulting public outcry and political uproar ultimately led to the 1994 division of the BGA into three successor institutes.[81] Just as in the past, however, the incident did not activate possible lines of cleavage between "insiders" and "external" critics. Decision-making procedures at the newly formed Bundesinstitut für Arzneimittel- und Medizinprodukte (BfArM) thus mimicked previous BGA approaches. Even though the spread of AIDS and concerns about drug approval rates were important features in German politics of the 1980s and early 1990s, comparatively little pressure was put on the network of physicians, regulators, and the pharmaceutical industry.

Likewise, industry-sponsored initiatives to change European Union laws prohibiting the advertisement of prescription drugs to consumers have made little headway because of opposition from the medical profession and government health ministries. As strong contributors or even primary payers of health care, governments fear that satisfying a "consumerist" European patient will greatly increase expenditures on pharmaceuticals. In a recent report, advocates of direct-to-consumer advertising nevertheless foresaw changes, in part because they anticipate the consumerist model will supersede current definitions of the patient: "Between 41% consumers (in France) and 57% of consumers (in Germany) generally support DTC [direct-to-consumer] as a concept for patient empowerment."[82]

Constructing the Patient in Drug Regulation

Regulatory interventions in the United States and Germany during the twentieth century demonstrate two alternative methods for pursuing drug safety and efficacy. Differences between the FDA's control of premarket testing and the BGA's control of market authorizations reflect authority struggles among the medical profession, pharmaceutical industry, and regulatory agencies. Debates about new legislation are key to understanding each nation's therapeutic culture, especially when dissimilar constructions of "the patient" and visions of the "consumer" were at stake. In the United States, reformers advocating greater, or less, government oversight mobilized competing visions of the patient. In Germany, debates centered on professional authority and ways to maintain a network for decision making that distributed authority among industry, the BÄK, and the government. This system proved resistant to change—even when confronted with patients visibly harmed by drugs such as thalidomide—primarily because no organized opposition challenged physicians' duty and right to speak for the ill.

The relative importance of consensus also differed in the two countries. In the United States, collaboration among industry, physicians, and the state was comparatively unimportant, since new laws and significant regulations were enacted largely in response to drug disasters and protests by politically mobilized patients. During these windows of legislative or regulatory opportunity, existing proposals were modified quickly and introduced as evidence of the government's ability to mitigate the case at hand and prevent similar events in the future. In Germany, lengthy negotiations among key interests preceded the approval of new laws in 1961 and 1976. New legislation was enacted less in response to disasters such as thalidomide-induced birth defects than as a means by which the state could codify agreed-upon divisions of authority and stabilize the entire health care system.

Policy responses to harmful drugs in the two countries open another window into important features of their distinct therapeutic cultures. In the United States, the Sulfanilamide disaster and close call with thalidomide were widely seen as indicators of the state's failure to protect the public. Hence legislative reactions centered on expanding the FDA's authority and providing more reliable information to physicians. The lag between the appearance of thalidomide-induced side effects and approval of a law granting the German government control over drug testing illustrates how the division of regulatory authority and responsibility among the state, industry, and the medical profession narrowed the inclination of any one group to use the disaster for political ends. Visible state-centered responses to this and other disasters were comparatively unimportant in the German political context.

Consequently, drug laws passed by legislatures in these two countries embodied different negotiations over the status, rights, and identity of patients. Precautionary regulations passed in the United States in 1938 and 1962 came out of the context of protecting the public from mislabeled or harmful drugs and guarding "guinea pigs" from unethical testing. Access to medicines first gained political saliency with the rise of disease-based activism in the 1980s. German drug laws after World War II first mandated a registration process, then instituted drug safety and efficacy requirements. Despite the relative absence of "the patient" from debates among the BGA, industry, and the medical profession, these organizations found their interests converging in providing sick Germans with rapid access to drugs.

The relevance of these two settings for regulatory decisions became visible in debates over how quickly medicines were approved for patient use. Both premarket control and postmarket study produce health risks for patients as well as political risks for the regulatory system. On the one hand, regulatory decisions based on extensive premarket testing require government agencies to accept accountability for withholding potentially life-saving drugs from patients. This option appealed to American regulators because of a therapeutic culture characterized by an advanced degree of critical external observation and politicized relationships among industry, the FDA, the medical profession, and disease-based organizations. On the other hand, regulatory decisions based on postmarket control require government agencies to accept the risk and accountability for possible adverse effects of a drug that is approved too rapidly. German physicians, industry, and the BGA were willing to accept this potential outcome because of a political context characterized by long-standing relationships among organizations in the network and a low degree of critical external observation.

Drug laws and regulatory interventions feed back into changes to each country's unique therapeutic culture. While therapeutic cultures evolve over time, Germany has repeatedly defended the promise of universal care. As part of that tenet, ill people were defined in relation to group membership, the potential for lost productivity, and general risks to the "body politic." In the United States, by contrast, debates raged concerning an individual's right to health care, public versus private boundaries in medicine, and the degree to which patients should be protected from industry and the medical profession as unwitting "guinea pigs," or given information as free-market "consumers." Contrasts between these two therapeutic cultures are also apparent in the more localized context of clinical trials, which form the topic of the next two chapters.

3

Clinical Trials from Treatment to Test, 1950–1980

CLINICAL TRIALS ARE CENTRAL TO THE PRODUCTION of knowledge about a drug's effects on humans. In order to promote the "objective" clinical trials required by American and German drug laws, physicians and regulators in the two countries seek to shield testing from industry influence and overtly political manipulation. Therapeutic cultures nevertheless manifested themselves in the inner workings of clinical trials. This chapter describes how American and German therapeutic cultures influenced the testing and regulation of Terramycin (an antibiotic), thalidomide (a sedative), and propranolol (a heart medication). The case studies in this and the following chapter—which examines interleukin-2 (a cancer treatment) and indinavir (an AIDS drug)—illustrate that drug testing differed in the two countries. In the United States, a quest for objective drug assessment led the FDA to demand multiple controlled clinical trials and statistical evaluation of their results. In Germany, an analogous quest for test results free from unseemly influences led government officials and the medical profession to promote qualitative testing methods and to collaborate on the review of smaller clinical tests. This contrast in approaches to testing emerged from their therapeutic cultures, most notably as a response to different constructions of "the patient" that prevailed between 1950 and 1980.

In each country, relations among the state, industry, medical profession, and disease-based organizations shaped the relative importance put on research and treatment during clinical trials. This quartet of actors interacted in complex ways during trials and in later evaluations of the outcomes. As we shall see, clinical trials serve not only a medical purpose of determining drug safety and efficacy, but also a political one of mediating among conflicting knowledge claims, divergent social expectations, and competing views of expertise.

During the early post–World War II era, key actors in both countries found their interests converging on greater use of clinical trials.[1] For government regulators, data from trials could narrow the field of decision-making choices by characterizing drugs primarily in terms of their safety and effectiveness. Pharmaceutical companies found that testing helped target populations who would purchase a new drug, generated information useful in marketing, and raised the entry costs for new firms seeking to market competing products. Medical reformers and consumer protection advocates expected premarket tests to prevent harmful or useless products from reaching consumers. For all these actors, clinical trials ultimately became intertwined with the public display of their professional and managerial competence.

Yet there are important differences between testing practices as they evolved in the United States and Germany. These center on clinical trials as sites for negotiating issues of demographic representation, determining the political authority of medical professionals, and mediating relations between industry and the state. Physicians' authority over the clinic came under attack in both countries during the period covered here. Nevertheless, opposition to the notion of individual patients as "cases" for scientific study in Germany ultimately shored up expert authority. In the United States, the imposition of uniform testing procedures and expectations for a standardized "patient" ultimately weakened physicians' professional authority.

Physicians and FDA officials in the United States used trials to establish professional boundaries among medical disciplines and develop the basis for official regulatory decisions. Clinical trials evolved as a management tool to select patients likely to benefit most from early exposure to experimental drugs and identify populations at risk from adverse reactions. Regulators found formal standardized testing procedures helpful as a shield against criticism and a means to respond to public concerns about drug safety. In Germany, on the other hand, trials were an important means for physicians to define their authority in relation to the state and establish new professional norms for medical care. Clinical trials carried out in the period between 1950 and the mid-1970s thus were integrated into overall patient care, rather than forming distinctive sites of professional and public debate.

Differences between the two therapeutic cultures are particularly apparent in exchanges among government officials, company representatives, and physicians about the results of clinical trials. Mechanisms for exchanging information differed, most visibly in publications describing experimental methods and testing results. Clinical trials initially offered doctors in both countries a means by which they could share information about new medications. Physicians worried throughout the twentieth century that medicine lacked a rigorous scientific underpinning. Greater comparability of test results, it was hoped, would support the use of successful therapies and eliminate harmful ones. In the United States, the FDA's strong regulatory presence resulted in the transfer of test results to regulatory and political arenas beyond the confines of the medical profession. In Germany, on the other hand, the greater authority vested in the medical profession allowed physicians to communicate almost exclusively with one another in medical journals, conferences, and informal discussions.

Two intertwined elements were put in place between the early 1950s and the late 1970s to facilitate dissemination of the results of clinical trials in each country. First, clinical pharmacologists learned to "raise the world," just as Pasteur had done by moving from laboratory testing to field trials of vaccines in the nineteenth century.[2] In other words, physicians in each country worked outside the confines of medical clinics to configure political and economic arenas where testing results answered questions about how best to treat disease and resolved controversies about health care spending and allocations. Second, the medical profession enforced a sufficient degree of standardization on individual trials and written reports to allow for comparison among them. Physicians had to devise a common structure for clinical testing that would leave sufficient play for the introduction of new techniques and allow for disease-specific experiments.[3] Nevertheless, differences emerged between the two countries traceable to their medical and regulatory traditions. As shown in the case studies, debates in the United States about proper methods for testing drugs between 1950 and 1980 track a decline of professional authority and expansion of FDA control. Greater cooperation among key actors in the German regulatory network during the same period guaranteed the medical profession a more significant role in drug regulation.

Origin Stories for Clinical Trials

Medical practitioners and historians have traced the origins of clinical trials to biblical accounts of dietary comparisons under Nebuchadnezzar II, James

Lind's study of scurvy on sailing vessels, and Edward Jenner's reports of small-pox vaccinations in the 1790s.[4] These individual cases, however, are perhaps best understood as interesting anomalies, rather than as a progressive lineage leading inexorably to contemporary methods of drug testing. Anglo-American and German proponents of clinical trials diverge when describing the emergence of their profession in the twentieth century. Whereas Austin Bradford Hill is often cited as a founding father in England and the United States, German clinicians attribute modern methods for drug testing to Paul Martini, a professor and physician at the Bonn University Clinic. Neither Martini nor Hill immediately changed the practices followed by a majority of physicians. Over time, however, their ideas and methods would come to play important roles in the evolution of clinical trials as very different policy tools in the United States and Germany.

Three clear contrasts between the two countries emerged in clinical testing during the 1940s and early 1950s. First, cross-disciplinary exchanges and collaboration allowed statisticians to gain a foothold in, and then increasingly dominate, the professional discourse on drug testing in the Anglo-American arena. In contrast, German physicians largely maintained and even expanded their disciplinary authority to define methods and practices employed in clinical tests. This led to a second difference in the emphasis put on selection criteria, treatment and control groups, uniform dosage regimens, and "objective" diagnostic tests such as laboratory analysis of urine or blood. Statisticians in England and the United States put great emphasis on each of these, irrespective of the disease in question, while physicians in Germany typically recommended using diagnostic and testing methods specific to the disease at hand. Third, authors describing testing methods in England and the United States stressed the "scientific" presentation of results, while German authors only rarely addressed issues of data presentation or writing style.

Hill had the opportunity to apply his ideas shortly after World War II when he helped design experiments with the antibiotic streptomycin on tuberculosis patients. Sponsored by the British Medical Research Council (MRC), this clinical trial's use of concurrent controls was later praised as "ushering in a new era of medicine."[5] The statistician Hill and his medical colleagues at the MRC used streptomycin's extreme scarcity and expense as a justification for allocating patients into treatment and control groups through a process of formal randomization. In doing so, they hoped to eliminate a form of "treatment bias" whereby physicians tended to select healthier patients for an experimental medicine than those receiving a placebo. The streptomycin trial was intended as a step toward "double-blinded" trials, in which neither researcher nor patient would be able to differentiate between treatment and placebo. Above and beyond the scientific rationale, random selection also allowed organizers to avoid difficult moral choices regarding which patients would receive the new therapy.[6]

At roughly the same time as the streptomycin trial in England, physicians and government regulators in the United States turned their attention to experimental design and methods of data analysis. FDA scientists seeking to implement the 1938 Food, Drug, and Cosmetic Act published articles in medical journals describing proper clinical trial methods, and the agency took an active role in promoting standards for drug testing during and after World War II.[7]

In contrast to the formal networks emerging among physicians, statisticians, and government officials in England and the United States, drug testing in Germany remained under the exclusive control of the medical profession. Unlike Hill, who had a background in statistics, Paul Martini was first and foremost a clinician. Consequently, his influential monographs on "Methods for Therapeutic Investigations" neither referenced statistical works nor invited statisticians to contribute to drug testing.[8] Nevertheless, Martini advocated greater use of mathematical techniques and formal testing of new therapies. He disparaged physicians who based their findings on a small number of case histories. Reflecting concerns found among German research physicians, he also recommended "blinding" procedures to minimize the impact of "suggestion" on recovery. In effect, Martini wanted to integrate new testing methods with existing therapeutic practices and so to defend the clinic as a domain controlled solely by the medical profession.

Despite important similarities in the methods they advocated, Hill placed greater emphasis on formal experimental design, while Martini sought to retain flexibility with respect to the specifics of different diseases. Hill and his North American colleagues, including Harry Gold at the Cornell Medical School, mapped out general criteria for drug testing and specified the stages that each trial should follow. According to physicians seeking to make medicine more scientific, patients were to be selected through formal criteria and then randomly separated into treatment and control groups. During the trial, clinicians were enjoined to employ techniques of double-blinding, use "objective" technologies for diagnosis, observe subjects at uniform intervals, and vary drug doses according to a planned schedule.[9] Only with proper planning, reformers believed, could trials produce reliable quantitative outcomes. Specifically, advance planning by physicians and statisticians was necessary to select a disease for a trial and specify criteria to judge success or failure. The new methods were intended to apply regardless of the specific disease. Hill's program thus aided a broader agenda of therapeutic reform by shifting the methods and focus of medical research from categorizing individual disease histories to measuring the impact of therapeutics across a variety of diseases.

Like Hill and his American colleagues, Martini wanted to advance scientific medicine by devising testable hypotheses. He also wanted to prove that select therapies worked in order to dismiss those that did not: "The closer we get to a truly causal therapy, the more generally effective treatments will become."[10] In order to prove a relationship between a new treatment and a patient's recovery, Martini suggested that physicians should first collect baseline measures, then experiment on patients divided randomly into treatment and control groups. He advocated blind tests (*unwissentliche Versuchsanordnung*) with placebos that were identical to the experimental drug in their form, color, and taste. In order to minimize the influence of confounding variables such as the "disposition, immune response, psychological status, age, sex, social and economic situation, and race" of patients, Martini compared large numbers of subjects in the test and control groups.[11]

Nevertheless, he did not want to fully ostracize confounding factors from medical study. For example, he noted that large patient groups were rarely available to test treatments for acute diseases. Martini also gave attention to specific methodological issues arising from the treatment of chronic diseases and suggested that physicians should collect individual case histories for each patient. Martini thus sought to develop a general theory for statistical evaluation of new therapeutics while retaining attention to individual patients and their specific ailments.

Although quantitative analysis of cases was seen as a sign of progress toward rational scientific medicine in the United States, German physicians were leery of this practice after World War II. Defining the individual patient as a mere case, an example, or a statistical value was too easily associated with the horrors of the Third Reich. Alexander Mitscherlich, an official delegate of the Federal Chamber of Physicians (Bundesärztekammer) to the Nuremberg physicians' trial, drew a powerful association between seeing patients as cases and atrocities carried out by physicians: "Only in the crossing of two currents could the doctor turn into a licensed killer and publicly employed torturer: at the point where his aggressive search for truth met with the ideology of the dictatorship. It is almost the same thing to see a human being as a 'case' or as a number tattooed on his arm."[12]

Christian Pross and other contemporary German historians of medicine have argued that Mitscherlich had relatively little impact on his colleagues in the early postwar years. Even though the German medical profession ignored or even actively repressed its Nazi past, the issue of a medical case as something other than an individual was contentious in the late 1940s and 1950s. Unlike their American counterparts, German doctors feared the replacement of the individual patient's unique circumstances and disease history by a standardized "subject" needing uniform care. In their documentation of the Nuremberg trial, Mitscherlich and his colleague Fred Mielke argued, "Overall it has shown how humanity and medical sovereignty perish when a science only sees people as objects and treats them as such."[13] Reacting to international outrage and emerging postwar moral sensibilities in Germany, physicians purposely avoided using placebos and double-blind experiments on new drugs.

Unlike the preoccupations of physicians in England and the United States with quantitative testing methods, German doctors first wanted to anchor the medical profession as a self-governing field with ethical standards based on the Nuremberg code.[14] A striking example of the shift in physicians' professional identity after 1945 can be found in passages from 1938 and 1947 editions of an introductory medical textbook, *Die Heilkunde und der ärztlichen Beruf.*[15] Whereas the earlier text posited National Socialism as the basis for a uniquely German medical practice, the postwar edition instead suggested that the medical profession provided physicians with an international cosmopolitan outlook.[16] Martini further illustrated this shift in a 1953 speech, when he suggested that the medical profession should observe the whole patient and even entire populations in order to validate specific disease therapies.[17] The German medical profession acted in concert to claim authority over the clinic, thereby preventing statisticians from making the same inroads as in England and North America.

Physicians in the United States and Germany developed different research designs and followed diverging approaches when testing drugs in the late 1940s and early 1950s. Though both defined scientific testing as involving random division of subjects into comparable treatment and control groups, as well as the use of statistical measures to quantify patient responses to therapies, the authors of key methodological treatises differed in ways that helped define American and German therapeutic cultures. In the United States, formal trial designs, an emphasis on quantification, and extensive precautionary testing were gradually institutionalized, whereas German testing methods reflected greater qualitative analysis and reliance on clinical observation of specific disease conditions. As Harry Marks has argued, clinical researchers in the United States conceived of controlled clinical trials before they had the social authority and organizational structure to carry them out.[18] In Germany, organizational concerns took a back seat to the focus on rebuilding the medical profession as an autonomous social group after the disaster of the Nazi period. This contrast, namely between reliance on formal process on the one hand and dependence on informal professional expertise on the other, would become embedded in regulatory structures and the institution of clinical trials during the following decades.

Case 1. Terramycin: The Era of Wonder Drugs

American and German clinical trials in the 1950s similarly relied on qualitative observations of patients, despite efforts by medical elites to institute quantitative methods. This was the case for penicillin and a series of other antibiotics including streptomycin, Aureomycin, Chloromycetin, and Terramycin. Following penicillin's wartime introduction and rapid canonization as a "miracle drug," each new antibiotic was announced to the medical profession with progressively larger advertising campaigns. In the United States, cooperative agreements between industry and the government characterized penicillin's wartime development.[19] Within a few years, however, collaboration gave way to intense competition among drug companies, and penicillin's price slipped from $20 to 2 cents per dose. As Pfizer's president John McKeen remarked, "If you want to lose your shirt in a hurry, start making penicillin and streptomycin."[20]

Nevertheless, Pfizer and other pharmaceutical companies envisioned a profitable future selling other antibiotics. Starting in 1947, Pfizer scientists screened some 100,000 soil samples collected around the world by missionaries, foreign correspondents, airline pilots, and other travelers.[21] Within two years, the company had identified an antibiotic in soil taken from Terre Haute, Indiana. Soon named Terramycin, the drug was shown to have low toxicity in animal and human tests. Perhaps equally important, Terramycin's potential to treat a broad spectrum of infectious diseases offered Pfizer the opportunity to market it as a direct competitor to antibiotics available from American Cyanamid (Aureomycin) and Parke-Davis (Chloromycetin).

Terramycin in the United States

Clinical tests on the new compound started in New York City in late 1949. Shortly thereafter, the firm distributed Terramycin to physicians in over one hundred hospitals and clinics around the country. Walsh McDermott, a physician with expertise in antimicrobial drugs, soon reported curing a recalcitrant case of pneumonia. After compiling success stories of treating diseases ranging from pneumonia to chronic diarrhea, Pfizer filed a new drug application (NDA) with the FDA at the end of February. Agency officials raised concerns about the drug's safety based on their review of the animal studies. Medical officers soon were convinced by the company's response and allowed the application to proceed.[22] By the end of March 1951, Pfizer had launched an extensive advertising campaign and begun mass production of the drug. During the next two years, the company spent $7.5 million promoting Terramycin and was the single largest purchaser of advertising space in the *Journal of the American Medical Association* (*JAMA*) between 1952 and 1956.[23] Pfizer submitted additional applications for a variety of forms and dosages, including pills, powders, intravenous, and eye drops. By 1952, American physicians could prescribe Terramycin for nearly forty distinct medical conditions, ranging from asthma to whooping cough.

Terramycin's rapid development and testing were typical for antibiotics at the time. Physicians recruited for clinical tests integrated it into their regular medical practice. Formal techniques of randomization, blinding, and use of placebos as advocated by statisticians such as Hill were not yet in widespread use. Nevertheless, doctors did pay close attention to diagnostic methods, compiled and tabulated their observations of patients' responses to the drug, and employed a progressive approach to testing dosages on patients. Different clinical trials of Terramycin followed very similar testing protocols and physicians reported results in a similar format. Publications from clinical tests carried out before the drug was approved contained detailed descriptions of testing methods and analytical approaches. These publications offer a window through which we can observe the testing practices of the time.

In the initial round of studies, physicians eagerly tried the drug on patients with nearly any infectious disease. They therefore used varying numbers of patients in each study and typically did not pick participants based on uniform criteria. For rare ailments such as Rocky Mountain spotted fever, some physicians even lamented the limited number of patients available on whom they could try out the new therapy.[24] The use of small groups—most of the tests had fewer than fifty participants—allowed doctors to study each patient carefully when testing Terramycin. Physicians tested the drug against a large number of diseases in their patients, and even used it to treat patients with multiple infections. For example, one publication described treating fifteen patients whose conditions ranged across the medical spectrum, and included pneumonia, streptococcal infections, subacute bacterial endocarditis, and urinary tract infections.[25] Larger studies tested Terramycin on ten or more different diseases, but did not include controls. Likewise, even large studies did not employ blinding techniques. Instead, both patients and physicians knew who was receiving the experimental drug. This lack of controls or blinding fits with Ortho Ross's contention in 1951 that only 27 percent of clinical trials were "well controlled," compared to 45 percent that had no control groups.[26]

Publications describing Terramycin's clinical use were rich in details regarding its impact on individual patients. By providing the kinds of information most useful to other practicing physicians, authors addressed concerns other than the methodological issues of interest to Martini and FDA officials. American physicians instead granted supremacy to concise but thorough descriptions that incorporated details of the patient, the disease, and the treatment regimen. For example, the recovery of a young woman suffering from a heart infection and paralysis on the left side of her body led to the following report:

> Case J.S., age 19, female. . . . This patient, the growth of whose *Staphylococcus aureus* was inhibited by 2.0 mg. / cc. of Terramycin, by 4 un. / cc.

of penicillin, but not by 5.0 mg. / cc. of Chloromycetin, was admitted on February 8, 1950, severely ill and semicomatose, on the ninth day of disease, after having failed to respond to intermittent treatment with sulfadiazine and penicillin at home. Terramycin therapy was instituted on the 11th day of illness and continued for 53 days. Progressive gradual improvement ensued. . . . At the time of discharge on the 59th hospital day, recovery was apparently complete.[27]

Published case histories combined precise measures of a disease and the exact treatment regimen with more qualitative assessments of the healing and recovery process. Descriptions of the course of a disease document that physicians observed their patients closely and noted changes, however small. Other doctors reading these reports could then compare them to their own past experiences with a given disease. They then considered published results in light of individual cases that they confronted in hospitals and private practices. This strategy to transfer results from the clinical trial to broader field practice relied on a large body of professional knowledge as well as physicians' ability and willingness to apply lessons from other case histories when treating their own patients.

Case descriptions also made up the bulk of the application Pfizer filed with the FDA, and government officials even assisted in their production. Ernest King, a medical officer at the FDA, was listed as first author on a *JAMA* article describing clinical success with Terramycin less than two months after he evaluated the Pfizer application.[28] He would later approve a number of additional Terramycin formulations. Likewise, Henry Welch, director of the FDA's antibiotics division, treated cases of chronic diarrhea in 1949 with "Combiotic," an otherwise unidentified Pfizer experimental drug. The report he sent to the company mirrored published case studies in its attention to clinical detail:

> *Case 7.* The patient was a white woman, age 32, whose chief complaint was a persistent diarrhea of five year's duration with five to twenty stools daily. . . . The common therapeutic measures including large doses of penicillin and streptomycin parenterally gave no or temporary relief. . . . The patient was given Combiotic tablets, two in the morning and two in the evening for six days. Improvement was noted after twenty-four hours and the condition cleared up in forty-eight hours.[29]

Welch's involvement with the clinical testing of medicines that he also reviewed as an FDA official became a scandal in the late 1950s, and he was forced to resign from the agency.[30] John Lear, science editor of the influential *Saturday Review*, was particularly disturbed by the income Welch had earned from reprint sales as editor of several medical journals.[31] Indeed, Welch's personal profiteering while in government service would become the main point of contention for reformers of drug regulation, largely eclipsing questions about his testing methods and drug approval decisions. More generally, cozy relationships between drug companies and regulatory officials came under fire as evidence of the "capture" of public interests by industry.

Terramycin's testing and regulatory approval in the United States offers a baseline against which to measure later changes. Medical experts tested this new medicine using largely qualitative techniques of patient observation and employed progressively stronger doses until patients recovered. FDA officials took reports from clinical studies at face value and allowed Terramycin's marketing mostly on the basis of personal contacts. Even though the 1938 Food, Drug, and Cosmetic Act had granted regulatory authority to the FDA, medical officers needed to draw on a network of physicians and company officials in order to carry out their mandate. Close contact with the industry, however, was widely perceived as contrary to the public interest, and officials would feel obliged to demonstrate their independence by the early 1960s.

Terramycin in Germany

Similar close ties among industry, physicians, and government officials emerged gradually in the fledgling Federal Republic of Germany during the late 1940s and early 1950s. Unlike the case of streptomycin in England, limited supplies of Terramycin did not induce German physicians to design formal clinical trials with random allocation of patients into treatment and control groups. Instead, Terramycin was integrated into postwar practices of close physician-patient interactions much like those found in the United States. While its scarcity posed special ethical dilemmas regarding who would obtain the drug, neither German physicians nor government officials sought to institute a rigid testing regimen as a rationing technique. Employing more of a free-market approach, physicians negotiated directly with suppliers and individual state health ministries to obtain supplies of the potentially life-saving antibiotic.

Initial German-language reports of Terramycin's potential as an antibiotic simply summarized American laboratory, animal, and clinical tests.[32] Beginning in 1951, the drug was imported by Boehringer Ingelheim under a licensing agreement with Pfizer. The company then initiated a series of clinical trials by sending the drug to select German physicians. Terramycin shipments, however, were often interrupted by transportation difficulties or held up by customs officials in these early years. To ameliorate supply problems, Pfizer established a production site in Brussels in 1953.[33] The company eventually built a plant in Germany in 1961 and then terminated its production arrangement with Boehringer.

Boehringer officials repeatedly negotiated supply issues with the German Interior Ministry, then responsible for granting permits necessary to market Terramycin. Company scientists provided ministers with medical descriptions of the drug, arguing that it was a powerful antibiotic against a variety of bacterial and protozoan diseases. Nevertheless, economic factors dominated discussions between the company and government officials. Boehringer, for example, cited difficulties with the availability of the *Deutsche Mark* and unpredictable exchange rates when ministers questioned the company's decision to import and then dilute strong Terramycin dosages. Company officials also requested a standing import permit, seeking to avoid the need to file for a new one with each shipment.[34]

Correspondence from 1951 documents the difficulties faced by Boehringer in obtaining sufficient U.S. dollars to import some 4,000 packages of Terramycin each month. In March and April of that year, the government only allocated enough U.S. currency to pay for 1,645 packages. In order to increase imports, the company offered to use its own currency reserves from export sales. Boehringer then had to document Terramycin's "advanced therapeutic value" in order to establish "the urgency of its import."[35] Individual medical practitioners were enrolled as part of these efforts. Physicians combined reports of Terramycin's safety and effectiveness with requests for increased supplies in letters written both to the company and to federal and state ministers.

Like their American counterparts, German doctors used Terramycin on small numbers of patients, generally fewer than thirty at any one time. Because of supply problems, many physicians could only try out the drug on two or three patients at a time. Doctors complained to the Interior Ministry that they would have preferred to test more patients, in order to give "the necessary weight to our publications."[36] Boehringer even included physicians' requests for more Terramycin when documenting its safety and efficacy to the government:

This case concerns a chronic *E. coli* infection of the urinary tract in a 65 year old male that has been present for 12 years and induced a constant, considerable impairment to his overall well-being, and led to attacks of fever and hypochromic anemia. . . . Tests of the infection revealed that the bacteria were nearly completely resistant to Sulfonamide, penicillin, Streptomycin, and Aureomycin. . . . The response to Terramycin, however, was astonishing. . . . Unfortunately, we only had sufficient supplies for two days. . . . We would be most appreciative if you [Boehringer] could supply us with additional dosages in such instances.[37]

As in the United States, German physicians used Terramycin against a wide variety of diseases, even within the same study. Because of its scarcity, the drug was reserved for serious infections during the early 1950s and was not prescribed as a substitute for penicillin or sulfa drugs. Physicians thus observed patients carefully and developed detailed case histories of Terramycin's effect on patients suffering from a range of life-threatening infectious diseases.

Clinical Approaches in the 1950s

Clinical studies carried out in both countries during the early 1950s employed advanced techniques to identify, diagnose, and track disease progression in patients. Methods included the use of X-rays, blood analysis, and urine analysis. German physicians employed stronger dosages of Terramycin than their American counterparts, while often worrying that they would run out of supplies. Letters to the company and the Interior Ministry warned of potential disease resistance from switching patients to weaker antibiotics.

Terramycin and most other antibiotics in common use during the 1950s produced mild side effects, if any. As a result, physicians on both sides of the Atlantic increasingly believed that modern pharmaceuticals were free of adverse reactions and that testing procedures and government policies were adequate and appropriate. Hill, Martini, and other reformers—including FDA officials—wanted drug tests to separate patients into experimental and control groups and employ techniques of single- or double-blinding. Once the sedative thalidomide was linked to thousands of birth defects in the early 1960s, reformers in both the United States and Germany found they had new authority to force change in pre-clinical testing and clinical trials. In the United States, this would come about through greater government oversight of the pharmaceutical industry, while in Germany the medical profession would expand its control over these areas.

Case 2. Thalidomide: Lessons from a Disaster

Starting in 1959, parents and physicians in Europe, Australia, Japan, Brazil, and elsewhere suddenly encountered a wave of children born with abnormalities. Defects grouped together under the heading "phocomelia," from the Greek for "seal limbs," included stunted arms and legs, misshapen hands and feet, and damaged internal organs. Because of diminutive long bones between the hand and shoulder or foot and hip, children's hands and feet appeared to grow directly from their torsos. Previously identified in the medical literature as an extremely rare condition, cases were rapidly on the rise in pediatric clinics.[38] By the time thalidomide was identified as the culprit and the drug was withdrawn, some 10,000 deformed children were born around the world. Between 4,000 and 5,000 of these births occurred in Germany alone, while the United States registered only 17 cases, born to mothers who carried the drug back from travels or were given it as an experimental treatment.[39]

Thalidomide's initial development and testing offered few indications that it would be a potent teratogen. Synthesized in 1953, the compound was first tested in university clinics and then marketed across Germany starting in 1957 by Chemie Grünenthal, a small chemical and pharmaceutical firm.[40] As a treatment for insomnia, tension, and even nausea associated with pregnancy, it offered a breakthrough in terms of safety. Unlike barbiturate sleeping aids, accidental overdose or even intentional suicide appeared impossible with this new drug. According to some reports, adults had taken up to four grams at once without adverse reactions, far exceeding the recommended 50 to 100 milligram dose. Patients reported that it induced a very pleasant sleep with few after-effects. Although not tested on pregnant women in medical clinics, it was used to mitigate morning sickness during the early stages of pregnancy. Consequently, Grünenthal marketed the drug to men and women in Germany with ads depicting peaceful nature scenes and suggested using thalidomide as a break from stressful work life. The company also developed international markets by exporting the drug and selling it under licensing agreements, making it available in over forty-six countries by 1960.[41]

Contergan in Germany

Grünenthal's advertising campaign proved successful and Contergan, the German trade name for thalidomide, was the top-selling sedative in Germany by 1960. Its sales of DM 12.4 million were five times those of the leading competitor.[42] According to one estimate, some 700,000 Germans took it on a regular basis. Parents even gave it to their children, earning Contergan the nickname, "West Germany's baby-sitter."[43] Adverse reactions were relatively rare, though some users complained of tingling in their extremities—a feeling that their arms and legs had gone to sleep—that persisted even after they stopped taking the drug. Nerve specialists Ralph Voss and Horst Frenkel reported some of these "peripheral neuritis" cases with the company, but Grünenthal officials showed little interest in following up on their findings once animal tests proved inconclusive.[44]

Beginning with informal conversations at the 1960 meeting of the German Society for Pediatric Medicine, several physicians began to suspect that Contergan also was causing the rash of birth defects noticed in clinics around the country. One of these, Widukind Lenz, a pediatrician and university professor, emerged as an active participant and spokesman for the medical profession in debates about possible links between Contergan and birth defects. Like other pediatricians, Lenz was surprised by the sudden appearance of phocomelia among infants born in his clinic. When he accepted a newly created chair for Human Genetics at the University Hamburg in 1961, he turned his full attention to these cases and began compiling detailed reports from his own patients as well as from other clinics in the area.[45] Within a short time, he had collected case reports from thirty-nine children that he linked to Contergan.

Lenz first reported his findings at the 1961 meeting of the Society for Pediatric Medicine. Even though he was growing convinced of Contergan's causal role in birth defects, he did not name the drug in his talk on 18 November. Nevertheless, his presentation attracted a large audience and was covered in the 26 November issue of the *Welt am Sonntag*, a weekly paper with broad circulation across the country. While the newspaper also did not mention Contergan by name, it did report that "a frightening increase in deformities has occurred in recent years" and recommended an immediate withdrawal of the dangerous medicine.[46] The same week, officials at the Federal Health Office brought Lenz together with Grünenthal representatives for a six-hour meeting concerning Contergan's market status. Company officials disputed Lenz's data and even succeeded in having him removed from the room for part of the meeting. Although Grünenthal continued to contest Lenz's findings behind the scenes, the company withdrew Contergan from the German market on 27 November.

During the next year, Lenz and other physicians gradually accumulated and analyzed further evidence linking Contergan to birth defects. Their early publications relied exclusively on individual case studies and noted the association with Contergan as tenuous. For example, in a January 1962 *Lancet* article, Lenz claimed that he had observed over fifty cases. In addition, he invoked a network of contacts in Germany, Belgium, England, and Sweden to claim 115 cases in which Contergan was thought to be the causal agent.[47] Subsequent articles demonstrate a shift from individual case reports to animal studies and aggregated data sets. These publications contrasted rates of birth defects among children whose mothers took Contergan with those who were not exposed to the drug. Consensus on Contergan's effects thus was built using comparative data and invoking vaguely the concept of a controlled epidemiological study—itself a controversial topic in the early 1960s.

At the same time, clinical tests carried out in the mid-1950s before Contergan was on the German market came under retrospective scrutiny. A public uproar and controversy regarding Contergan's testing, even among experts, led to disputes concerning nearly every aspect of drug testing. When physicians and pharmacologists looked back at early tests with the drug, they frequently expressed dismay with research methods. One of the first to argue this point publicly was Wolfgang Heubner, a pharmacology professor at the University of Heidelberg. In an article in *Der Spiegel*, he observed that "the present, all-too typical approach, whereby a practicing physician gives out a new drug and then reports on the 'favorable' results in a medical journal a half year later simply does not suffice."[48] Grünenthal's failure to oversee testing more carefully and the readiness with which the company accepted and spread the claim that Contergan "lacks any toxicity" ultimately undermined the company's explanation of its testing and marketing practices.

Scientists and managers from Grünenthal had to defend their decision to market Contergan in court when federal prosecutors filed a 972-page criminal indictment in 1967. After spending five years compiling and evaluating 70,000 documents, they claimed that Grünenthal had marketed a harmful product and that company officials failed to act when told of adverse reactions in 1959 and 1960. In what would become an even larger undertaking, some 2,000 statements were read into the public record as 120 witnesses and 60 experts provided testimony and underwent cross-examination over the course of 283 court days. Even though the indictment was filed against eighteen Grünenthal scientists and managers, by the time the trial ended in December 1970, only seven were still present. The others either had passed away or been dismissed for medical reasons.[49]

Trials of this magnitude are unusual in the German legal system, since judges typically maintain strict control over courtroom proceedings by preventing lengthy disputes over evidence, limiting the number of motions attorneys may file, and appointing expert witnesses directly.[50] The Contergan trial ended only when prosecutors dropped the criminal charges in exchange for Grünenthal's agreement to establish a fund for the injured children. Created with an infusion of DM 150 million—100 million paid by the company and 50 million by the federal government—the fund remains active to this day. As part of the settlement, the company and individual defendants were released from further criminal or civil liability.[51]

Prosecutors called upon several clinical investigators during the trial to describe tests they had carried out on the medication prior to its marketing. As became abundantly clear to the judges and courtroom observers, few of the investigators had conducted systematic studies. Instead, physicians had relied heavily on patients to assess the drug and were often only vaguely aware of more rigorous testing approaches advocated by Paul Martini and other medical reformers. For example, Franz Heinzler, a physician at the University Clinic in Düsseldorf, testified that in 1955 he had given Contergan to patients in the evenings as a sedative and then asked them about its efficacy. This vague description, however, did little to satisfy the judges:

Vors. [chief justice]: What you just said is too little for me. I would like to hear from you whether a specific plan was established?
Dr. Heinzler: No, that wasn't done.[52]

In subsequent questioning, Heinzler offered few specifics on testing procedures, how many patients he observed, or for how long his patients received the then-experimental drug. He did testify that discussions with colleagues had led him to believe Contergan had no lethal dosage, making it a good alternative to barbiturates. Consequently, Heinzler gave the drug to any patient who complained of a lack of sleep or felt restless. Under steady questioning by the judge, Heinzler recalled a daily dose ranging from 50 to 100 milligrams. He claimed familiarity with techniques of control groups and placebos, but when prodded by the judge admitted that he had not employed them in his clinic.

When queried about adverse reactions, Heinzler stated that he had not paid them any particular attention, and could not recall any complaints. The judge then asked a series of questions about a 1956 publication in which Heinzler described his research findings. In particular, the judge noted that the publication described placebo use and precise testing methods. Heinzler, however, could not verify that the procedures he himself endorsed had actually been followed, stating simply that "I did not see any side effects of a serious nature in the stationary patients, and other than some constipation, I simply did not observe anything."[53]

In contrast, when the physician Karl Otto Vorlaender was called to the stand some ten days later, he readily conceded that Contergan was not tested using rigorous methods like those recommended by Paul Martini, his director at the Bonn medical clinic. Vorlaender considered his tests a pre-clinical study to determine if the drug was worth examining further in a "precise" clinical trial. Testifying to the court, Vorlaender expressed regret that "this large clinical trial did not take place" as a follow-up to his research.[54] In the study he did oversee, Vorlaender followed Martini's dictum to only test one medication at a time. He therefore excluded patients who were already on other medication. Of 600 patients he treated each month, only 80 to 100 fit this definition, since those with "serious" stress-related conditions received barbiturates.

Turning to the dosage regimen, Vorlaender explained that he had developed a standard protocol, first taking patients off other drugs, then stating to each, "Please take a tablet of this substance K17 tonight and report the results to me in the morning."[55] He recorded results for each patient and compiled specific findings in detailed patient histories. Concluding in 1957 that Contergan was an effective therapy, he nonetheless shifted his primary research interests to immunology and did not carry out a larger trial. As Vorlaender testified in the trial, Martini would have demanded strict controls and a rigid trial design necessitating time and resources unavailable to Vorlaender. After Martini re-tired in 1959, the Bonn clinic's involvement with Contergan faded, especially when the new director heard about its association with nerve damage.

These two witnesses—Heinzler and Vorlaender—offer a good indication of the range of methods used in German clinical testing during the 1950s and early 1960s. On the one hand, Heinzler relied primarily on casual contact with patients and sought to obtain an overall sense of how well the medicine worked for a variety of patients, including people taking other medications. On the other hand, Vorlaender gave only Contergan to his patients and then inter-viewed them individually as to its effects. Furthermore, he carefully tabulated results in patient histories, intending to design a more systematic study. Yet the differences between Heinzler and Vorlaender were themselves contained within a set of professional practices common to clinical testing across Ger-many. Physicians had sole authority over the design and structure of the trials. They did report results to the manufacturer and often published findings in journals, but no government authority or other professional association re-viewed methods or outcomes.

Although methods followed in clinical studies of Contergan became a central part of the court case and were widely reported and debated in the press and medical journals, few significant changes can be traced directly to the incident. Some experts even disputed the necessity of structural changes to clinical testing. For example, when drawing lessons for pharmaceutical com-panies, one analyst argued, "The immediate responsibility for carrying out clinical tests lies exclusively with the testing physician."[56] According to this view, companies should review the credentials of physicians selected to carry out clinical trials, but should not interfere with testing methods. The govern-ment likewise had no role to play in the clinic. Professional associations ul-timately stepped into this void and issued formal recommendations for clinical trials.

Despite the outcry and publicity generated by the Contergan tragedy and the lengthy court case, few demands arose for greater government oversight or structural reform in German clinical trials. Notably, the government was not blamed for its lax oversight of the drug market. Instead, the monopoly position of the medical profession to speak for "the patient" held steady despite the very visible tragedy of Contergan-induced birth defects.

Thalidomide in the United States

In striking contrast to the situation in Germany, and even though far fewer children were born in the United States with thalidomide-induced deformities, regulatory laws were strengthened and clinical trials underwent significant changes. The U.S.-based pharmaceutical company William S. Merrell, Inc., signed an agreement with Grünenthal to license the drug for the American market in 1958. Following initial toxicology and pharmacology tests, broader clinical trials started in early 1959, and continued for twenty months with few reports of adverse reactions.

The company's testing campaign incorporated elements of mass marketing when Merrell sent samples to over a thousand doctors, suggesting they give it to any patient complaining of stress or having trouble sleeping. Merrell was so confident of thalidomide's safety that the firm used its investigational drug status as a means to enroll physicians and build brand-name loyalty to the medicine. According to FDA tabulations made in 1962, nearly 16,000 patients, 624 of whom were pregnant, took the drug in its investigational phase.[57] Through good fortune, most women received the drug after the first trimester, and only seventeen phocomelic children were born in the United States.[58]

Concluding that the drug was as safe for the American market as it appeared to be in Europe, Merrell submitted a new drug application for "Kevadon," thalidomide's intended American trade name, in September 1960. At the time, the FDA employed seven full-time and four half-time medical officers to deal with roughly 300 human and 150 veterinary new drug applications each year. Officials reviewed applications primarily on the basis of materials provided by manufacturers. The criterion that a new drug must be proven safe for use in a specific indication did not require the FDA to carry out experiments of its own. In most cases, reviewers did not have the time or resources even to carry out extensive literature searches. Officials had sixty days to voice their objections; otherwise a new drug was considered approved.

Medical officers working for the FDA were aligned with other reformers of the late 1950s and early 1960s in their desire for more rigorous clinically controlled drug testing. Consequently, the agency adopted a skeptical stance toward the methods employed in clinical tests and sponsors' exaggerated claims. Nevertheless, agency officials were not expected to pass judgment on the clinical value or effectiveness of new medicines, making it difficult for them to challenge testing methods common to the medical profession.

The presumed easy review of a sedative with few side effects and low toxicity was assigned to the newest FDA employee, Frances Kelsey. While new to the agency, she had years of experience with drug testing stemming from her research on anti-malarial compounds during World War II. Kelsey also had helped edit an introductory text on pharmacology, first published in 1947 and revised in subsequent editions.[59] As a result, she had a solid background for evaluating the thalidomide application, which included data from 3,156 patients grouped into fifteen trials.

Kelsey and two other reviewers—a chemist and a pharmacologist—each found deficiencies in the initial application and explained their objections in a letter to Merrell. They questioned the completeness of animal data and methods used to determine the identity, strength, quality, and purity of the drug.[60] Furthermore, as Kelsey wrote to the company, "The chronic toxicity data are incomplete and therefore, no evaluation can be made of the safety of the drug when used for a prolonged period of time."[61] In a report to her supervisors, Kelsey argued that the application was "rather superficial" and expressed doubts that thalidomide would find a "useful place in therapeutics."[62] Kelsey and her colleagues looked at every aspect of the application and demanded additional data regarding thalidomide's impact on animals and humans. Their communication put the application on hold. A new sixty-day deadline for FDA review would be initiated only when the company responded with supplementary laboratory and clinical findings.

Over the next several months, Merrell first complained to the agency about Kelsey's requests, but then submitted additional information.[63] While reviewing the revised application, Kelsey and her colleagues noticed a letter in the *British Medical Journal* linking four cases of peripheral neuritis to thalidomide use.[64] When queried by Kelsey, Merrell's scientists responded that the incidence was extremely low and rapidly reversible. But to Kelsey and outside consultants including Raymond Bieter, a pharmacologist from the University of Minnesota, the peripheral neuritis cases suggested they exercise extreme caution with the drug. In turn, the company argued that Kelsey's recruitment of outside experts was unjustified and indicated that she was overreaching her authority.

Responding to Merrell's criticism of her actions, Kelsey drew a strong line between her regulatory role and the company's responsibility for testing: "In the consideration of an application for a new drug, the burden of proof that the drug causes side effects does not lie with this Administration [the FDA]. The burden of proof that the drug is safe—which must include adequate studies of all the manifestations of toxicity which medical or clinical experience suggest—lies with the applicant."[65]

By delineating the difference in obligations between a company conducting drug studies and the FDA reviewing final data, Kelsey was also staking a claim for the government over the clinical domain. The agency would only approve drugs when tests followed rigorous methods and generated "proof" of safety. Unlike German physicians such as Lenz, Heinzler, or Vorlaender, who tested drugs and made safety determinations that substituted for government regulatory decisions, Kelsey did not need to design medical experiments or establish causal evidence. Nevertheless, government officials like Kelsey could specify what kinds of tests would meet the "burden of proof" that a new drug was safe.

Kelsey's critical stance regarding the clinical testing of thalidomide followed from the agency's goal under the 1938 law to standardize and compare even individual subjective experiences with new therapies. Merrell's debates with the agency over what counted as proof of safety, however, suggest that many physicians and company executives were unfamiliar with new testing methods in this area. FDA officials and reformers such as Henry Beecher, the physician famous for exposing unethical experiments on human subjects, felt that individual symptoms and subjective responses to treatment could be quantified through better methods.[66] For example, Beecher had published a textbook suggesting that even pain, the most subjective of all patient experiences, could be quantified. He recommended controlling variables through experimental designs that would "standardize the activities of all subjects prior to medication."[67] Physicians in different clinics could then observe and study patients using the same set of measures to evaluate the performance of an experimental drug. For a sedative like thalidomide, clinicians could use a standardized reporting form to query patients about the drug's effects.

Despite Merrell's pressure on her to approve the drug, Kelsey repeatedly postponed a final decision on thalidomide by requesting additional tests during the spring and summer of 1961. If anything, pressure from the company to approve the drug hardened Kelsey's stance on the need for long-term toxicity data and formal clinical trials. In addition, the FDA's status as a centralized regulatory agency gave her a basis for making these demands, unlike individual crusading physicians such as Lenz or Vorlaender in Germany. Once the tragedy in Europe drew intensive media attention, reports in the United States lionized Kelsey and pointed to the success of the FDA review process in preventing thalidomide from gaining market approval.[68]

Merrell withdrew its application in early 1962. The FDA then investigated the company's testing procedures and found instances of falsification and failure to submit data. For example, close comparison of actual lab notebooks with materials in Merrell's NDA revealed that some dogs identified as receiving thalidomide had instead received sugar, changes had been made to autopsy reports, and the company had scaled rat growth curves to its advantage.[69] The drug's wide distribution as part of "investigational study" then came under harsh criticism from journalists such as John Lear of the *Saturday Review*.[70]

Officials also carried out a massive campaign to destroy all remaining thalidomide tablets. Warning that the pills were "still at large in family medicine cabinets" and could easily be mistaken for other drugs, the FDA contacted physicians who received thalidomide from Merrell and asked the public to "flush unidentified drugs down their toilets."[71] To FDA officials, "The drug firm clearly was not conducting research but engaging in a practice popularly known as 'seeding the marketplace.'"[72] The product recall further aided the larger FDA agenda of reforming testing methods. By making an example of Merrell and by writing and phoning some 1,200 clinical investigators, government officials hoped to change how companies and physicians ran tests in the future.

The Changing Clinical Setting

Events associated with thalidomide in Germany and the United States eventually became the starting point for a new round of debates over drug safety, requirements for proof of efficacy, and reforms of testing procedures in each country. In the United States, thalidomide gave additional momentum to physicians and regulators who wanted to reform testing practices by introducing placebo controls and double-blinding techniques to clinical trials. As described in the previous chapter, it stimulated a rapid legislative response. Once the 1962 Kefauver-Harris Amendments were passed into law, the FDA issued regulations spelling out acceptable testing methods. Companies that failed to follow FDA rules faced the possibility that their medicines would not gain market access.

In Germany, the thalidomide disaster instead helped cement the authority of the medical profession to issue guidelines and determine qualifications necessary for running clinical trials. Rather than demand the introduction of quantitative testing techniques, physicians instead recommended careful observation of patients and longer periods of data gathering. As this difference in their therapeutic cultures indicates, very different political demands and expectations were placed on clinical trials in the two countries. Nevertheless, in both countries political and medical authorities found greater clinical testing an ideal method to control market access for new medicines.

Case 3. Propranolol: Taking Drugs "For Life"

Following the thalidomide disaster, clinical trials of drugs for chronic conditions increasingly focused on the presence of adverse reactions, even among small numbers of patients. Unlike antibiotics, which are generally taken for only a brief duration, medicines for heart conditions, central nervous system disorders, or diseases such as diabetes are taken for indefinite periods. As a contemporary Novartis advertisement suggests, these drugs must be taken "for life."[73] The same pills that reduce pain for people suffering from angina pectoris, mitigate arrhythmic heart beats, or help treat hypertension can also become a less benign "life sentence" that requires patients to adhere to strict dosage regimens, live with uncomfortable side effects, and pay for multiple drug prescriptions.

Beta-blockers, drugs that prevent the uptake of adrenaline by heart and chest cells, illustrate some of the promises and risks posed by long-term therapy to individual patients, regulatory agencies, and the medical profession. Tensions arose in both the United States and Germany regarding the ability of relatively small and short-term clinical trials to uncover side effects that would only become apparent in larger populations that took a drug for a long duration. Different approaches to testing and regulating new drugs in the two countries led to contrasts in the importance placed on finding side effects before drugs could be marketed. In the United States, regulators demanded extensive testing to identify precisely which adverse reactions would affect which patient population. In Germany, the medical profession adopted a more lenient perspective on initial approvals but relied on postmarket studies to modify prescribing practices and reduce cases of adverse reactions. Striking contrasts thus emerged between the two countries in requirements for the certainty of disease etiology, proof that a therapy worked beyond the power of physician suggestion, and the ability to predict and manage side effects before allowing a drug on the market.

Heart pain, cardiac insufficiency, and arrhythmic heartbeats are among the most complex and culturally variable diagnoses known to modern medicine. Ever since William Heberden characterized chest pain with an "ominous prognosis" as angina pectoris in the late eighteenth century, disputes have raged over angina's underlying physiological pathology and appropriate treatment measures.[74] While some medical practitioners considered angina pectoris to be simply the "phenomenology" of chest pain as described by patients, others sought to find causal "pathophysiological processes" that would clarify links to other heart conditions.[75] The late-nineteenth-century view that angina resulted from restricted blood flow led to the use of amyl nitrite and nitroglycerin in Europe and North America. Both compounds helped to relax smooth muscles, thereby easing patient complaints. Research carried out in England during the 1950s by James Black, a scientist at Imperial Chemical Industries (ICI), demonstrated that beta-blockers such as propranolol could inhibit the uptake of adrenaline by heart and chest muscles. This prevented painful muscle constrictions.

German and American conceptions of the heart and heart pain, however, differed in ways that had a profound impact on the introduction of the beta-blockers in the 1960s and 1970s. In Germany, the "lingering influences of romanticism," to borrow Lynn Payer's apt characterization, promoted a less mechanical view of the heart than in Anglo-American medicine.[76] German physicians rarely associated different disease profiles to the heart alone, linking them instead to patient complaints ranging from poor circulation to depression. The heart was considered part of a nuanced and complex circulatory system that has a variety of possible pathologies, including coronary insufficiency (*Herzinsuffizienz*), weakness from age (*Altersherz*), and angina pectoris.[77]

Pain associated with angina was evidence of a constriction in the blood vessels, making vasodilatation a popular therapeutic approach.

In the United States, on the other hand, angina was thought to result from a physiological disturbance in the surface of the chest wall or in the ribcage. Physically distinct from the heart, anginal pain was not viewed as predictive of heart attacks (myocardial infarction). A clear distinction was drawn among arrhythmic conditions, angina pectoris, and myocardial infarctions, with different therapeutic approaches recommended for each diagnosis.[78] Of the three, angina was viewed as the most problematic for rational therapeutics, particularly since subjective patient reports were the only data available to judge a drug's efficacy.

Beta-Blockers in Germany

Animal and human tests of Dociton, propranolol's German trade name, began in the early-1960s, shortly after ICI marketed the drug in England. In 1965, Rhein-Pharma, the German licensee for the compound, registered Dociton with the Federal Health Office (Bundesgesundheitsamt, or BGA) and began distributing information and advertisements to physicians. Dociton's testing, regulatory review, and marketing in Germany illustrate remarkable physician autonomy in the division of the regulatory terrain among government, industry, and doctors. Materials submitted by Rhein-Pharma in order to register the new drug consisted largely of physicians' reports. The company did not reevaluate clinical studies and government officials offered no challenges to claims about the drug's safety.

In materials sent to physicians, Rhein-Pharma readily acknowledged that early beta-blockers, in particular Alderin, had caused powerful toxic reactions in patients. Dociton, according to the company, had the same level of toxicity, but was ten times as efficacious. Patients therefore could take significantly weaker doses and would not suffer from side effects.[79] Evidence used in Germany to support the drug initially came verbatim from tests conducted in England. Within a few years, the British studies were complemented by reports in German medical journals that described both individual case histories and structured trials of Dociton. Even though the Rhein-Pharma brochure suggested that side effects were of a "fleeting character," German physicians stressed the need to observe patients closely. Rather than seek a standardized dosage, they urged one another to customize each patient's dosage in order to prevent serious adverse reactions.[80]

Side effects of beta-blockers, later a crucial point of debate between regulators and company representatives in the United States, thus were by no means ignored in Germany. Government officials, however, tended to place great faith in voluntary reporting systems run by medical commissions. The Federal Chamber of Physicians (Bundesärztekammer, or BÄK) had assumed responsibility for collecting data on side effects during the 1950s and 1960s. In a 1969 article, the BÄK's Drug Commission (Arzneimittelkommission der deutschen Ärzteschaft, or AkdÄ) argued that the American approach to determining therapeutic efficacy was overly rigid. According to their perspective, the overemphasis on scientific experimentation in the United States excluded drugs from the market whose efficacy was evident from long-term use by practicing physicians.[81] In addition, German physicians criticized the American focus on "routinized" tests as interfering with the development of new testing methods. Reports of side effects from beta-blockers, including skin problems, shortness of breath, and headaches were therefore interpreted as indicators of the need to modify an individual patient's dosage. Such reports were not taken as prima facie evidence of the need to carry out formal clinical trials.

Balancing risks and benefits from beta-blocker therapy was considered the province of physicians alone. Publications describing the results of clinical testing therefore emphasized that "the risk of iatrogenically induced *Herzinsuffizienz* must constantly be weighed against the danger or harm posed to the patient from their primary condition."[82] Risk calculations were not, however, based solely on qualitative measures of patient performance. German physicians were extremely precise in monitoring the pulse and blood pressure of patients complaining of heart problems. When they put patients on Dociton, heartbeat patterns were charted before, during, and after drug therapy.[83] Published illustrations displayed "regular" and "irregular" heart patterns, showing significant changes in individuals taking beta-blockers. Improvements to the "chamber frequency"—a measure of irregular or fluttering heartbeats—ranged from 9 to 44 percent over the course of four to forty-five minutes.

This kind of variation drove FDA officials to distraction when they encountered it in the American new drug application. In the German clinical setting, variation from one patient to the other was more acceptable, if not always expected. German medical experts who evaluated Dociton's safety and efficacy accepted reports specific to individual patients that included few data points amenable to statistical comparison. Indeed, Germany's therapeutic culture supported decision making that relied on informal expert assessment rather than formally designated criteria for test results.

Acceptance of statistical uncertainty when offset by patient recovery contributed to the use of combination therapy in Germany. Physicians prescribed Dociton alongside older treatments for angina, such as Amyl Nitrates. Even after Dociton had been on the market for eight years, a 1973 review essay admonished physicians to begin therapy by treating behavioral and lifestyle factors such as obesity and smoking. They should next couple beta-blockers with other medications.[84] Combination therapy in a predetermined sequence was common in Germany by the early 1970s. Even though some studies of combination therapy—especially of propranolol with Amyl Nitrate—were carried out in the United States, they drew more attention in Germany than in North America.[85]

By 1974, speakers at the German Society for Internal Medicine advocated the use of beta-blockers for a variety of conditions. The University of Munich medical professor Helmut Lydtin began his talk by suggesting that "every practicing doctor" should be aware of beta-blockers' usefulness in treating hypertension.[86] Lydtin further argued that beta-blockers were now so well understood that they could become part of "standard therapy" for high blood pressure and angina. Nevertheless, he warned his colleagues that they should design individual dosage regimens and observe patients closely for adverse reactions.

Lydtin's warning was borne out in the side effects produced by the beta-blocker Practolol. Problems with this drug first appeared in individual case reports published in the *Lancet*. These documented serious eye effects, often coupled with a skin condition resembling psoriasis. After the publication of several reports, two hundred additional cases of eye damage were reported to the British Committee on the Safety of Medicines, some of which were nearly three years old.[87] In response, ICI-Pharma, the German division of ICI, contacted physicians in Germany and asked them to report any problems with Practolol to the Drug Commission.[88] By November 1974, commission leaders had collected reports of thirty-nine serious adverse reactions in Germany, including six cases of conjunctivitis and twenty-eight of psoriasis-like skin damage.[89]

Practolol's removal from the German market, however, proceeded only through a laborious series of discussions among the company, the BGA, and the Drug Commission. After several inconclusive meetings, a "deutsch-englisches Experten-Meeting" was called in March 1975 to decide on Practolol's future.[90] Following this conversation among company representatives, British and German regulators, and officials from BÄK's Drug Commission (AkdÄ), the company withdrew Practolol from the general market. It did remain available to hospital clinics upon request. AkdÄ also published warnings telling physicians to stop prescribing the drug.[91]

The testing, registration, and ongoing discussion over the safety of beta-blockers in Germany illustrates the stability of networks of trust among physicians, industry, and the government through the mid-1970s. Propranolol's rapid marketing after only a small number of studies had been completed in England and started in Germany was based on assurances from the company that this drug was safe. Its use was nevertheless circumscribed by physicians' caution in administering potent heart medications. Practolol's withdrawal due to adverse reactions was a carefully orchestrated event that prevented public outcry and maintained physician authority over patients. In Germany, the BÄK operated as the central node in a web of relations among patients, physicians, drug companies, and government officials. Since physicians individually controlled prescriptions, and the medical profession as a collective governed market access and drug withdrawals, little pressure was mounted to change testing methods and introduce greater quantification to the clinical setting. Likewise, the boundary between premarket testing and postmarket review was more flexible. In effect, Dociton gained rapid market access precisely because it was under constant observation and testing.

Propranolol in the United States

In the decade following the 1962 Kefauver-Harris Amendments to the Food and Drug Act, the FDA increasingly understood its regulatory mandate as one of clearly separating drug testing from marketing. This required the agency to insist upon strict scientific criteria and mobilize a network of experts to stake out its position. The FDA's separation of test from market operated much like a "boundary" between science and society that sociologists have characterized as a "contextually contingent and interests-driven pragmatic accomplishment."[92] Government regulators adopted a cautious approach when granting market approval to a new drug by reviewing its application carefully and insisting on rigid clinical trial design. Propranolol's testing thus took place in a period when FDA officials were seeking to instill norms of placebo use, double-blinding, and statistical analysis of results among physicians testing experimental drugs. Doctors interested in getting access to innovative medicines and trying them on a broad spectrum of patients were slowly forced to follow clinical trial methods that incorporated experimental and control groups and other aspects of formal testing.

Ayerst, the American firm that licensed propranolol from ICI, went through nearly ten years of correspondence and meetings with the FDA in order to get the drug approved for treatment of angina pectoris. Inderal, as the drug was named for the American market, was approved to treat arrhythmic heart conditions in 1967, but not for angina or hypertension. When the company put together a separate application for angina pectoris, FDA officials turned it down. In a lengthy letter explaining their decision, medical officers noted a series of design flaws in Ayerst's testing: inadequate pre-study observation, short treatment periods, a lack of uniform reporting systems or standard criteria for evaluating subjects, and too few patients in each study.[93]

Particularly troubling for the future of the propranolol application, the agency questioned the very notion of treating angina pain without curing patients of the underlying ailment. Explaining that the FDA took a dim view of any therapy that eased symptoms without correcting underlying causes, one official explained: "We have considered carefully the rationale of recommending a potent drug with many diffuse systemic effects and with potential severe side effects for the treatment of a symptom complex of variable etiologies."[94]

This medical officer argued that no drug could serve as a rational therapy if the sponsor did not narrow angina pain to a specific condition with a known etiology. In other words, the agency thought it unwise to use such a potent drug for a group of symptoms without a known cause. FDA officials wanted a single drug to treat a single disease, preferably without adverse reactions on the rest of the patient's body.

Cardiologists who had tested propranolol and found it therapeutically beneficial expressed their irritation directly to the agency. They also published articles on the issue, foreshadowing later debates concerning an American drug lag. For example, Albert Kattus, the chief of cardiology at UCLA, found the FDA referees incompetent to "make any judgment about a drug having to do with heart disease." In his experience, propranolol offered "the first true pharmacological advance in the medical management of angina since Dr. Lauder Brunton discovered nitroglycerin 100 years ago."[95] Kattus and a number of other cardiologists felt that the FDA's failure to approve propranolol was an unwarranted attempt to refute the diagnosis of angina pectoris and an inappropriate intrusion into their clinical domain.

Agency officials responded to these criticisms as well as to queries from Ayerst in an April 1970 meeting that brought together company officials, members of the Cardiovascular Advisory Committee, and cardiologists who had tested the drug. FDA medical officers started by again questioning the very concept of suppressing anginal pain, arguing that it served a useful warning to patients of underlying heart problems. Turning next to the data submitted by Ayerst, officials argued that five years of marketing experience in Europe did not equal well-controlled and well-designed clinical trials. Specifically, a government expert on statistics criticized the absence of baseline data, the use of multiple study designs, and the company's attempts to mask inconsistent measurements between studies. Particularly disturbing to the FDA, "much of the data is fundamentally subjective and it is not clear how it has been 'quantized.'"[96] In addition to concerns about the type of data in the propranolol application, medical officers from the agency raised questions about propranolol's safety, noting a high incidence of congestive heart failure.

FDA representatives thus went through a minute deconstruction of Ayerst's application. The company had submitted reports of eight controlled double-blind studies, involving 123 patients. Repeating criticisms articulated in the initial rejection letter, agency officials described inadequate pre-treatment periods, defective drug and placebo administration, failure to conduct pre-study observations, improper criteria for choosing patients, reports lacking details of the severity of individual attacks, and the use of other drugs during trials. This last point was significant, since unlike in Germany, FDA officials viewed combination therapy with great distrust. They argued that drawing cause-effect conclusions was nearly impossible when patients received more than one therapy at a time.

By discrediting Ayerst's application, FDA officers and members of the advisory committee were striving to standardize practices in clinical trials. They wanted companies to submit data of a more formal statistical nature, instead of relying on case reports. Company officials attending these meetings learned that they had to enforce comparability across different studies and had to lay the groundwork for statistical analysis by designing uniform testing procedures. Discussion on these points was often very specific. For example, when queried on how to maintain a double-blind study when physicians measured heart rates and discussed symptoms with patients, an FDA consultant suggested that "a fellow clinician not personally involved could make heart rate determinations and monitor patient management."[97] In denying Ayerst's propranolol application, FDA medical officers sought to use the company to change how doctors carried out clinical trials. The agency's detailed critique therefore eventually served as a template for designing clinical trials of propranolol.

Many physicians, however, resented this intrusion into their clinics. They regularly included in studies patients who did not meet entry criteria. At the same time, they defeated double-blinding methods by determining which patients were taking propranolol, often simply by observing heart rate changes. According to FDA criticisms, doctors also failed to gather sufficient background information on patients. They did not chart the severity of angina attacks, record the use of other medicines, or even note activities such as drinking tea or coffee that influence heart activity. For them, "the patient" was not a standardized input-output machine necessary for rational regulatory decisions. Instead, they saw patients as individuals who should be given medicine and care to promote recovery, or at a minimum, to reduce pain and suffering.

Regardless of physician resistance, Ayerst was forced to redesign propranolol's clinical trials several times in order to create a study protocol that would meet FDA requirements. For example, detailed negotiations were necessary to work out the entry criteria for a trial launched in 1973. The company wanted to accept patients who had two angina attacks per week, while the agency demanded five per week. Ultimately, both sides agreed that no more than one-fourth of any one test group could have fewer than five attacks per week. Restrictive FDA criteria for patient recruitment raised testing costs and extended the time needed for physicians to organize and carry out the clinical trial. The agency ultimately realized that it could not have a "pure" trial as its statisticians recommended, and compromised on the issue of recruitment. In other aspects, however, FDA officials held firm. For example, the company was not allowed to switch "non-responders" to another therapy, because the FDA felt such a move would hopelessly confuse the data analysis.[98]

In 1974, the Cardiovascular Advisory Committee met again to discuss propranolol. This time, members agreed that the company had documented the drug's efficacy in treating angina pectoris and that new clinical trials had shown the drug did not cause congestive heart failure. Nevertheless, the committee's support for propranolol was conditional on its use only for "moderate to severe angina in patients not responding to weight control, restriction of activity, cessation of smoking, and use of sublingual nitroglycerin."[99] The American advisory committee members thus agreed with their German colleagues that a sequence of other interventions should be attempted before administering propranolol.

Within a few weeks of propranolol's approval, Ayerst again invoked the ire of FDA officials through advertising materials claiming the drug was the new "first choice" to treat angina pectoris.[100] The agency had only agreed to approve the drug as a third or fourth choice for patients still suffering after dietary and lifestyle changes coupled with nitroglycerin therapy. The FDA required the company to write every physician in the United States and inform them: "Inderal is an other than first choice drug for use in selected angina patients only after conventional measures have proven ineffective."[101] Having worked closely with the company in designing clinical trials, the agency also decided which trials could be cited in advertising and promotional materials sent to physicians.[102] In effect, agency officials not only imposed strict controls over the methods used for producing knowledge about propranolol, but also regulated the distribution of findings.

Regulating Clinical Trials in the 1960s and 1970s

Experiences with beta-blockers under the different review and evaluation systems found in the United States and Germany during the late 1960s and early 1970s illustrate some of the more general contrasts in how the two countries approached drug regulation. The FDA's gatekeeper role between testing and market gave it a position of authority when the agency negotiated with pharmaceutical companies over appropriate proof of drug safety and efficacy. This contributed to standardized clinical testing practices, but also led to time-consuming and politicized battles over trial design and analysis of results. The

German reliance on companies to engage trustworthy professionals for drug trials allowed for more rapid marketing of medicines, but simultaneously created the problem of having to later withdraw medicines shown to have serious side effects. In Germany, professional societies stepped in to monitor adverse reactions, but had to rely on voluntary reporting mechanisms to gather data about marketed drugs. Changes in testing methods were gradual and arose from within the medical profession. In contrast, changes imposed by the FDA were more radical in their nature and more rapid in their implementation, since companies had their very financial survival at stake in the testing and approval process.

A Regime of Numbers versus a Treatment Site

Clinical judgment and statistical authority persisted side by side in both the United States and Germany from the early 1950s through the late 1970s. In any one specific trial, they were either uncomfortably juxtaposed, or more commonly, one or the other was given greater weight. Medical elites in the United States who supported the use of quantitative clinical trials for therapeutic evaluation sought to replace clinical judgment, which they perceived as subjective and too easily influenced by pharmaceutical marketing techniques. Yet as the German case illustrates, clinical judgment remained a compelling basis for knowledge claims within the medical community—and continues to be so. Looking across the three case studies presented in this chapter, we see that increasing reliance on statistics in the United States was driven by the demands of a therapeutic culture that defined "the patient" as needing government protection from both industry and the medical profession. In contrast, Germany's therapeutic culture promoted a vision of "the patient" in need of physicians' professional guidance and support.

Discipline and Authority in the Clinical Trial and Beyond

The medical clinic and regulatory hearing serve as two key sites for power struggles among industry, the medical profession, and the state. Choices concerning the organization of clinical trials, participant / subject selection, and debates over appropriate outcome measures illustrate that medical and political aspects blended in both countries. In the United States, physicians, industry, and government officials all granted trials significant agency, and wanted them to provide uniform assessments of drug risks. They also used drug testing to establish norms for doctor-patient relations more generally. Trials offered physicians a way to communicate with industry and the state. In Germany, clinical trials remained a more flexible institution, reflecting greater stability in the medical profession and greater social consensus on the division of authority among the state, industry, and professions than found in the United States. Reports of drug tests remained largely internal to the medical community.

The degree to which clinical trials were thought of as "experiments" or as "therapy" differed strikingly between the two countries from 1950 to the mid-1970s. In the United States, drug testing was idealized as a controlled simulation of what would happen once a medicine came on the market, whereas in Germany treatment of patients in the clinic superseded efforts to set parameters on a drug's use. FDA officials and elite clinicians advocated quantified drug testing in America as a surrogate for the intimate knowledge and personal trust otherwise needed to share knowledge about disease treatments across physical distance and over time.

Government approval thus became, to borrow Bruno Latour's term, an obligatory point of passage before a new drug could reach the broader market. "Those who sit at this point, like Mercator [source of the geometrical map projection], carry the day."[103] In its position of power, the FDA could force companies to repeat tests until they met emerging government standards. Formal drug trials grouped patients into recognizable, disease-based groups and offered regulators a tool to publicly demonstrate their ability to protect patients from harmful or ineffective medicines. To that end, clinical trials transformed qualitative reports of doctor-patient interactions into quantitative data sets. The preference for quantification bred by America's therapeutic culture was reflected in new drug applications to the FDA and in published reports of clinical trials. Detailed descriptions of individual patients and qualitative analysis common during the early 1950s thus gave way to data tables, quantified measures of patient performance, and statistical analyses by the mid-1970s.

Greater integration of drug testing with regular therapeutic practice in Germany was reflected by publications on new drugs as well as in reports filed with the Interior Ministry in the 1950s and drug registrations at the Federal Health Office in the 1960s and 1970s. Physicians testing medicines in Germany relied primarily on qualitative methods to assess how patients reacted to new drugs. While the government exercised some control over the drug market, the medical profession could define testing methods and decide which drugs were safe without an additional point of passage before prescribing medicines to patients. Since German physicians had greater control over drug testing in the clinical setting than their American counterparts, statisticians made few inroads into these areas.

According to Ted Porter, who has written extensively on the history of quantification and statistics as a discipline, "The idea of a medical statistics was as old as statistics itself." Yet because of medicine's strong disciplinary identity and robust political authority, the "language of quantity" made few inroads until the middle of the twentieth century.[104] As Harry Marks has argued, the mathematical components of Hill's essays and textbooks, especially sections on means, variances, standard deviations, and tests of statistical inference, ultimately challenged notions of the infallibility of expert judgment. As the cases presented here illustrate, it required the FDA's engagement to convert clinical trials into a regime of numbers. In Germany, where the medical profession maintained its exclusive authority and the state had little regulatory power to force change, drug testing remained an area of qualitative expert assessment. These differences would themselves gain additional political salience in the 1980s and 1990s, when disease-based organizations challenged American regulatory norms and Germany more closely integrated clinical testing and drug regulation with the emerging European Union.

4

Clinical Trials as Test and Therapy, 1980–2000

DRUG TESTING UNDERWENT IMPORTANT CHANGES in both the United States and Germany during the 1980s and 1990s. Case studies of interleukin-2 (a cancer therapy) and indinavir (an AIDS drug) in this chapter illustrate a break in testing approaches and regulatory styles from an earlier period. Changes in the two countries arose from shifts in their therapeutic cultures. The American "patient" evolved from needing state protection from industry and physicians to a free-market consumer who deserved access to still-experimental drugs. As a consequence, the FDA placed fewer demands on manufacturers for lengthy testing and redesign of clinical trials as in the past. Advisory groups suggested that the agency instead monitor medicines more closely once they were on the market. German "patients" evolved in this period to require greater professional and state protection from modern biomedicine. The medical profession and government worked in concert to balance patient care and data collection in the clinical setting.

In the United States, further decline in the medical profession's monopoly to speak for patients contributed to the rise of disease-based activists and organizations that promoted a new politics of testing and care. These groups challenged the real world applicability of clinical trials that failed to adequately represent the diversity of final users. Criticisms were levied against such selection criteria as age and gender as well as exclusions for taking multiple medications or using alternative therapies. Activists considered strict scientific and regulatory standards for proving safety and efficacy unethical because of their reliance on placebos and refusal to inform patients whether they were in a treatment or control group. More generally, changes in the United States illustrate a renegotiation of authority and regulatory responsibility among the state, industry, the medical profession, and patients.

During the same period, implementation of the 1976 drug law in Germany consolidated authority over testing in the hands of clinical pharmacologists. Efforts to standardize testing and introduce quantitative techniques in the 1980s and 1990s were offset by the widely shared view among medical experts that patients, especially those with terminal illnesses, needed individual care and attention. The continued ability of the medical profession to speak for the patient in Germany meant that comparatively few tensions emerged between patients and the regulatory system. Instead, efforts focused on protecting patients from some of the excesses of modern medicine during premarket tests of new drugs. Disease-based activists posed few challenges to testing methods, and the network of medical elites, industry scientists, and government officials continued to determine drug safety and efficacy in much the same way as in earlier eras. German citizens did protest certain aspects of biotechnology; most notably challenging expert claims that genetic engineering posed few novel health risks. As the case studies document, their protests had little influence as drug review shifted from the German national setting to the European Agency for the Evaluation of Medicinal Products (EMEA).

Citizen groups mobilized differently in the two countries and had dissimilar impacts on clinical trials and regulatory decisions. In the United States, the presence of disease-based activists on the national political scene promoted important changes in the domestic policy agenda. Pharmaceutical drug regulation took on a more "postmodern" appearance when government officials recognized that definitions of safety and efficacy would necessarily vary depending on patients' backgrounds and the diseases they were fighting. Lacking the ability to represent the patient as a single entity in political debates over regulation, the FDA and the medical profession both acknowledged that clinical trials needed to include a demographic population representative of the country at large.

In Germany, critics also attacked trials for assumptions about the easy transfer of findings to the broader patient population. The focus of controversy in Germany, however, was on the failure of tests with new drugs to protect the rights of vulnerable individuals.[1] Clinical trials were faced with the difficult task of balancing scientific and regulatory criteria against historically grounded fears of medical experiments that failed to care for individual patients. Whereas the American medical clinic became a site for resolving issues of public access, representation, and equity, the German clinic became a front line for defending the "weak and sick" from well-intended testing with a variety of new biopharmaceuticals.

Citizen mobilization in both countries was coupled to demands for greater transparency and access to regulatory decision making. Testing regimes, previously designated as controlled and closed-off arenas, now needed to demonstrate publicly their political relevance and social acceptability. As in the past, debates over the results of clinical trials became intertwined with debates over the adequacy of methods. With additional actors, including disease-based organizations and other activists involved in these debates, drug tests were hard pressed to meet all the expectations. Outside groups increasingly expected to participate in judgments on a given drug's marketing status, not just hear about the final regulatory decision. As a result, procedures for making regulatory choices at the FDA, the German Federal Health Office (Bundesgesundheitsamt, or BGA), and EMEA evolved to incorporate broader definitions of acceptable data and flexible understandings of who counts as an expert.

Patients and disease-based organizations invoked local "subjective" experiences in an effort to offset the tendency of physicians and government officials in each country to focus solely on "objective" data sets. As we shall see, even though analogous criticisms were levied against scientific and medical expertise in both countries, the tension between clinical trials as a standardized testing site and a clinic treating patients played out differently in the United States and Germany. Their different therapeutic cultures thus produced not just different conceptions of research subjects and patients, but also influenced the formation and focus of new social movements.

Case 4. Interleukin-2: Biotechnology and the Market

In the mid-1970s, scientists at the U.S. National Cancer Institute (NCI) identified a set of compounds in the human body that appeared to control the immune system. Further research demonstrated that these "interleukins" regulate the production of T-cells, a class of white blood cells. Key to the immune system's ability to recognize and destroy bacteria and viruses, T-cells can also control and even eliminate cancers. Interleukin-2 (IL-2) was first isolated in the early 1980s, and scientists including Robert Gallo, later renowned for identifying the HIV retrovirus, were excited to learn that it encouraged white blood cell reproduction.[2] The ability to generate white blood cells in the laboratory, it was hoped, would revolutionize cancer research and therapy. Gallo and other NCI scientists expected that larger doses of interleukins would stimulate the body to destroy cancer cells without additional chemotherapy.[3]

Efforts to produce billions of white blood cells and then inject them into patients, however, were plagued by a variety of technical difficulties.[4] The treatment contained impurities, including remnants of T-cell cultures, interleukins extracted from animals, and other compounds. Patients responded poorly to the lab-generated cells and impurities. Small doses appeared to have little impact, while larger doses induced the immune system to attack diseased and healthy cells indiscriminately. A mid-range dosage produced dramatic results in some cases, but in many other patients, cancers did not go into remission or rebounded following the treatment.[5]

Concurrently, several new biotechnology companies also began exploring therapeutic uses for the interleukins. Scientists at Cetus, a small California biotechnology company, took up research in this area, backed by a wildly successful initial stock offering in 1981 that netted the company $115 million and set its market value at $600 million.[6] They soon began working on a therapeutic dosage of IL-2 as a means to bypass the problems created by laboratory-produced white blood cells. Company researchers expected direct injection of IL-2 to stimulate internal white blood cell growth with minimal adverse reactions. The compound, after all, was already present in the body. Cetus also hoped that internally produced T-cells would better differentiate between cancerous and normal cells.

Putting IL-2 on the top of its research agenda, the company increased production in order to start clinical tests. Whereas NCI scientists extracted IL-2 from mice spleens, using huge numbers of expensive rodents in the process, Cetus turned to recombinant DNA techniques for mass production. The company designed a strain of *E. coli*, a bacterium found in the human digestive tract, to carry the IL-2 gene. In order to distinguish their product from the IL-2 found in the human body, Cetus began using the name "Proleukin" for the recombinant version.

Once greater amounts of IL-2 were available, Cetus carried out in vitro and animal pharmacology tests. At the same time, the company worked with scientists at the NCI to begin human tests. Collaborations with NCI researcher Steven Rosenberg, perhaps better known for operating on President Reagan's colon cancer, led to cordial exchanges of raw materials and regular meetings to discuss interim findings.[7] In 1984, the company began clinical trials on humans, starting with 75 terminally ill patients. One year later, Rosenberg and his NCI collaborators began administering a "high-dose therapy" of IL-2 to ten patients.

Glowing cover stories in *Fortune* and *Newsweek* accompanied initial reports of the treatment's success in 1985. Warning that "cautious clinical investigators fear the familiar phrase 'cancer breakthrough' almost as much as laymen dread the word cancer itself," *Fortune* nevertheless stated that IL-2 could control a wide spectrum of cancers, and would perhaps cure all cancers. The article concluded, "Even if lymphokines live up to only half of their promise, there will be a lot of joyful faces—not only in the research clinics and in the board-rooms of companies well placed to profit from the breakthrough, but also . . . in countless households that the disease will touch."[8] *Newsweek* began its article similarly warning of the potential for a "wreckage of false hopes," but then claimed that a major breakthrough was imminent. The *Newsweek* article also suggested that techniques of "adoptive immunotherapy" would treat cancer bodywide, unlike more narrowly targeted surgery or radiation.[9]

Within days, over a thousand people had called the NCI cancer hotline, even though news magazines and television networks warned that results were preliminary and IL-2 was unlikely to cure every form of cancer. Coupled to the media exposure, Cetus's stock climbed from $14 to $40 per share. By the middle of the following year, the company had a market capitalization of over $1 billion, despite annual sales of only $50 million from diagnostics and no phar-maceuticals ready for FDA review.[10]

When NCI scientists published the results of their initial tests in *JAMA* the following year, the journal included an editorial critical of IL-2's side effects and extraordinary costs.[11] Two of ten patients in the NCI study had partial tumor regression, five were listed as "dead of disease," and the remaining three showed no change, or experienced slight additional growth of their cancers. According to Charles Moertel, a physician at the Mayo Clinic, the treatment was "an awesome experience" of long hospitalization and multiple visits to intensive care units. Furthermore, "the price in dollars for treatment and man-agement of toxicity may reach six figures. Such high human and financial costs demand commensurate therapeutic benefit."[12] According to Moertel, patients had few benefits, leaving the majority to suffer debilitating side effects. These included serious infections and capillary leak syndrome, a potentially life-threatening condition where plasma and proteins leak into the extravascular space. Capillary leak syndrome can produce heart attacks, respiratory prob-lems, gastrointestinal bleeding, and kidney damage. Nevertheless, Moertel's criticism of IL-2 therapy as too expensive and too toxic had little immediate impact on its further development by Cetus. The company proceeded to larger clinical trials in collaboration with the NCI, and by the late 1980s was ready to seek regulatory approval for Proleukin in the United States and Europe.

Although clinical studies reported by *JAMA* in 1986 offered a far more sobering assessment of IL-2's efficacy than found in popular magazines, it would take another two years for business journals to warn investors that the compound was not a "one-stop cancer breakthrough."[13] In the stock market crash of October 1987, biotech companies now criticized for relentless media hype and few marketable products saw their market valuations collapse. Entering what Robert Teitelman has characterized as the "iron age" of biotechnology, only cooperative research agreements, the sale of successful testing technologies, and licensing agreements with large pharmaceutical firms kept small companies fiscally solvent.[14] IL-2's revenue potential was assessed down to $275 million annually from as high as $400 million two years earlier. Nevertheless, Cetus and a couple of other firms sponsored over 80 clinical trials with recombinant IL-2 in the late 1980s. Even analysts critical of the hype regarding most anticancer agents anticipated a healthy revenue stream for this compound.

Proleukin in the United States

Before Cetus could begin earning money from Proleukin, it needed FDA marketing approval. By the time the time the company submitted a new drug application (NDA) for Proleukin to the agency in 1988, scientists had narrowed the proposed use to treatment of metastatic renal cell carcinoma, a disease affecting some 25,000 Americans per year. Cetus expected Proleukin to gain rapid approval for this indication, since it had a five-year survival rate of only 10 percent. When the FDA's Biological Response Modifiers Advisory Committee met to review the application, however, company hopes were dashed. Committee members requested additional studies and demanded that the company clearly specify which patients would benefit from the therapy. Cetus included results from studies on "metastatic cancer," but did not differentiate the source or type of cancers in its new drug application. The FDA Advisory Committee members were consequently not convinced of Proleukin's specific efficacy to treat kidney cancer.[15]

Two years later, the advisory committee met again to review a revised Proleukin application submitted by the company. Like their predecessors, advisory committee members requested that Cetus perform further research and carry out more specific data analysis. In particular, they challenged the selection of control groups, methods for compiling data, and, most important, the narrow selection of clinical trials for the new drug application (NDA). Cetus had attracted extensive publicity in the late 1980s with claims that it would soon cure a broad spectrum of cancers. Each of the many trials carried out on Proleukin, successful or not, drew media coverage. While necessary to the sequence of stock offerings that kept the company afloat financially, this media attention ultimately made it difficult for the company to justify its choice of studies when documenting Proleukin's efficacy in its NDA.

Widespread testing ultimately hurt the company since reviewers felt unclear about the dosage and precise treatment regimen advanced by Cetus. The advisory committee demanded that the company further clarify which patients were benefiting from Proleukin treatment. Furthermore, some members expressed concerns that the therapy required too much physician expertise and close patient observation. One committee member noted, "It may be fine in Steve Rosenberg's hands [at NCI] where he has a good staff to treat the side effects, or here at [Johns] Hopkins or other big places. But what about little hospitals? If this drug were widely used, we could see drug-related mortality go way up."[16] In effect, the advisory committee wanted a clearly specified treatment regimen that relied less on physician expertise and experience. Committee members acknowledged the importance of local skill and institutional experience with the treatment as key to its success. They were concerned that these prerequisites would translate poorly to other clinical settings.

After the advisory committee finished savaging the Proleukin application, Cetus's stock went into a predictable slide, eventually bottoming out at $8.75 per share a month later. Failure to gain FDA approval cut the company's market value by 75 percent to $276 million. Analysts speculated that parts of the company would be sold. Their predictions proved true when Chiron, a competitor located across the street in Emeryville, California, purchased Cetus for $660 million in 1991. As part of the deal, Cetus sold several patents, including the DNA replication system known as the polymerase chain reaction (PCR).

In order to prepare a revised application, Chiron focused on a smaller group of patients during an additional two years of clinical testing. Consequently, the 1992 application described just seven clinical studies with 255 patients, each of whom had metastatic or unresectable (not removable through surgery) renal cell carcinoma. Four of the seven studies were carried out at a single clinic, while the others were multiclinic trials. Three of the trials were of Proleukin alone, while the other four involved comparisons with treatments such as Interferon or injections of lymphokine-activated killer cells. No placebos were used, since patients were uniformly diagnosed with life-threatening cancers and FDA reviewers concurred with the lack of clinical controls or a double-blind. Proving Proleukin's efficacy and justifying the persistence of serious adverse reactions among most of the patients, on the other hand, were problematic for the company.

In the revised application, Chiron claimed that the duration of patient responses and stabilization of their ECOG Performance Status proved Proleukin's efficacy. The ECOG scale (Table 5), devised by the Eastern Cooperative Oncology Group, consists of five levels that gauge the influence of cancer on the "daily living abilities of the patient." ECOG, the largest of several American "Oncology Groups," traces its origins to NCI-sponsored clinical trials in the 1950s for leukemia treatments. By the early 1990s, it had grown into a largely autonomous clinical research organization.[17] For the Proleukin trials, ECOG's

TABLE 5 / ECOG PERFORMANCE STATUS

Status	ECOG
0	Fully active, able to carry on all predisease performance without restriction
1	Restricted to physically strenuous activity but ambulatory and able to carry out work of a light or sedentary nature, e.g., light housework, office work
2	Ambulatory and capable of all self-care but unable to carry out any work activities; up and about more than 50% of waking hours
3	Capable of only limited self-care; confined to bed or chair more than 50% of waking hours
4	Completely disabled; cannot carry on any self-care; totally confined to bed or chair
5	Dead

Source: Eastern Cooperative Oncology Group, "ECOG Performance Status," URL: ⟨http://ecog.dfci.harvard.edu⟩.

standardized table for patients' Performance Status (PS) served as a surrogate for more precise quantitative measures of responses to the treatment. When combined with the more easily quantified measures of tumor number and size, the performance status gave a well-rounded picture of patient response, albeit one reflecting the American conception of mobility and work activities as central aspects of patient health.

Of the 255 patients used for the revised application, 28 (11 percent) were classified as "partial responders," meaning that their tumors had shrunk by half or more, and existing lesions had not expanded in size. FDA officials were convinced by this measure of Proleukin's efficacy. They even reproduced Chiron's data in their Summary for Basis of Approval: "Seven of the 28 partial responders and none of the complete responders were symptomatic from their disease (PS=1) at study entry. Of these seven patients, one returned to baseline after therapy and the other six became asymptomatic (PS=0)."[18] Between the ECOG status and uncertainties in how to define "partial" and "complete" responses, proof of efficacy, now more than ever, required patient assessment and communication between physicians and patients in the clinical trial. Furthermore, the company and FDA officials had to negotiate appropriate measures of efficacy and how to scale data from various tests.

Proleukin's side effects continued to plague the application. Just as Moertel noted years earlier, the therapy was an "awesome experience" for patients who suffered damage to nearly every internal organ. Eleven of 255 patients died during the clinical trials, nearly half as many as experienced "partial" improvement. Once the drug was approved, the FDA published a two-page list of side effects, with detailed tables showing what percent of patients suffered damage to their cardiovascular, pulmonary, gastrointestinal, neurological, renal, hepatic, hematological, dermatological, musculoskeletal, and endocrine systems. Even a full week after therapy ended, some 14 percent of patients remained hospitalized.

As a result of the agency's further review of the application following the advisory committee meeting, the FDA insisted that package inserts begin with the stark warning: "Proleukin should be administered only in a hospital setting under the supervision of a physician experienced in the use of anti-cancer agents. An intensive care facility and specialists skilled in cardiopulmonary or intensive care medicine must be available."[19] As part of the eventual approval, the company announced that it would continue to monitor patients indefinitely to better measure Proleukin's long-term efficacy and safety.

Side effects—and Chiron's claim to be able to mitigate at least some of them through an extremely precise treatment regimen—had drawn close attention from the advisory committee. In a 1992 meeting, the committee recommended approval only under very specific conditions. Members endorsed a drug regimen under which patients receive Proleukin over the course of two five-day treatment cycles, separated by a rest period. Fourteen injections are given in each cycle involving a fifteen-minute intravenous infusion, followed by an eight-hour rest period. After nine days of rest, the schedule is repeated for another fourteen doses, for a total of twenty-eight doses per course of therapy.[20] Though ultimately convinced that patients could recover from side effects during the breaks, committee members still worried about the selection of patients for Proleukin treatment. In particular, they feared that patients with advanced cancers would be too weak to survive the therapy.

From a therapy intended to treat all cancers, Proleukin evolved in the course of clinical trials to a treatment solely for largely asymptomatic kidney cancer patients. Patients with an ECOG status greater than PS-1, that is, those most eager to get treatment, were denied the drug outside of clinical trials. Though the advisory committee's minutes hardly read like a ringing endorsement, the application soon earned FDA approval. Reporting on the decision, *Business Week* suggested that revenue would start slowly and climb to $100 million yearly, a sharp reduction from earlier estimates of a $500 million blockbuster drug.[21] By early 1993, over 1,000 patients had been treated with Proleukin, and Chiron proudly announced sales of $12.5 million, still far short of previous estimates.[22]

In its formal approval letter, the FDA demanded that Chiron obtain post-market clinical data in several areas. Although not a "conditional approval" per se, Chiron's promise to carry out additional tests and closely monitor patients following treatment clearly played a role in the FDA's decision to approve Proleukin. Specifically, the company agreed to obtain additional data on the duration of tumor responses and to examine factors that might help physicians predict how specific patient populations would respond to the drug. In closing out the summary for basis of approval in 1992, the FDA specified additional trials "required for licensure." These included additional animal studies as well as "investigation into patient characteristics which may identify patients likely to benefit from [Proleukin]," and "ongoing follow-up on tumor response and survival data from responders."[23] Chiron agreed to observe and continue treating patients who had participated in the clinical trials. In effect, as part of the deal struck to allow market approval, the company became responsible for long-term patient care.

One clear benefit to the company from sponsoring ongoing patient treatment and observation was demonstrated in 1997, when the FDA approved Proleukin for the treatment of metastatic melanoma. Based on a "retrospective analysis of patients" carried out to meet FDA requests for additional data, the company identified a cohort of 270 skin cancer patients who had responded positively to Proleukin.[24] In an initial review by the agency, the medical officer disagreed with expanding Proleukin's product license. Shifting rapidly from a statistical evaluation of efficacy to an assessment of side effects, the FDA reviewer argued, "From a statistical point of view, the data are inadequate to demonstrate that IL-2 provides a net benefit to patients with metastatic melanoma which outweighs the considerable risk. It is not enough to consider only the small number of patients who achieved a complete response under this therapy, without considering also the number of patients whose lives were adversely affected by this therapy."[25]

The agency's numerical weighting of harm from side effects as more significant than a small number of cures did not convince the advisory committee that reviewed Chiron's new application. Members instead emphasized that "metastatic melanoma is a disease that gives cancer a bad name," since it strikes young patients, progresses rapidly, and has extremely low long-term survival rates (only between 2 and 3 percent of patients survive five years once the disease is identified). While not perfect, Proleukin appeared to help 16 percent of patients. Out of 270 patients with melanoma treated between 1985 and 1993, 17 experienced a complete return to health and an additional 26 had a partial recovery. FDA representatives countered that this 16 percent response rate was offset by the 84 percent of patients who suffered severe adverse reactions without discernible benefits.[26] Advisory committee members nevertheless decided that the application merited approval, if accompanied by ongoing clinical studies. Reflecting a shift in America's therapeutic culture, committee members, like many of the patients they treated, were primarily concerned with providing reasonable access to the treatment. The agency, on the other hand, still faced political pressures to approve drugs with no or few adverse reactions.

At this point, discussion shifted to additional tests the advisory committee members expected in return for expanding Proleukin's approved uses. Committee members were deeply divided between suggesting "accelerated" or "traditional" approval. As one member noted, a full product license would give FDA officials little authority to demand additional clinical research. Accelerated approval, on the other hand, could be used to force the company to submit ongoing reports from clinics that observed and cared for patients after treatment.

During debates on how best to shape future Proleukin studies, concerns about adverse reactions mingled with consideration of the therapy's cost, even though drug prices are supposedly not a factor in approval decisions. Echoing the FDA reviewers, one advisory committee member argued, "We are talking about a very, very small number of patients that will receive a very, very toxic and extremely expensive therapy."[27] As an investigative report by the *Boston Globe* documented in 1998, the $45.9 million spent on Proleukin's development and testing by the NCI did little to lower its ultimate cost to insurers and patients.[28]

Despite concerns about its side effects and cost, the FDA ultimately approved Proleukin for metastatic melanoma, recommending a treatment regimen identical to that for kidney cancer. The agency again requested Chiron to monitor patients for at least five years after Proleukin therapy. Unlike the review of Propranolol in the 1970s, however, the FDA was now far more flexible about allowing a drug on the market despite evidence of serious side effects and limited statistical proof of efficacy. Clearly delineated boundaries between premarket trials and approval for widespread marketing had given way to a more flexible regime that allowed limited market access conditional upon long-term patient monitoring.

Biotechnology Policy and Politics

As described in the previous chapter, Germany developed a comparatively fluid approach to determining a new drug's marketing status between the early 1950s and late 1970s. The sharp boundary between clinical trials and postmarket surveillance found in the United States was never adopted in Germany, making the review of medicines such as interleukin-2 less stressful on the regulatory system. Whereas this drug's testing and regulatory review in the United States dragged out over a lengthy period, in Germany it proceeded comparatively quickly. At the same time, public concern with the human health and environmental risks posed by biotechnology prompted very cautious integration of the treatment into medical care. Published reports of clinical trials and documentation prepared in the company's application to the BGA consequently illustrate greater attention to risks to the health care system writ large and concerns about individual patient autonomy than in the United States.

Unlike the case-by-case review of biotech drugs and foodstuffs in the United States, Germany adopted a process-based regulatory approach marked by cautious assessment of risks to public health from recombinant DNA research and production methods.[29] Responding to public protests, federal and state regulations required firms to document not just the safety of their products, but also the physical containment of biological materials used in research labs and factories. Changes in the "Federal Nuisance Act" during the late 1980s required that effluent from industrial production facilities be completely free of microorganisms. Citizen groups concerned with biotech-based drug production agitated for additional government regulation and directly monitored company compliance with existing laws. They reported violators to government authorities and even sued manufacturers. As a result, production facilities, including BASF's Tumor-Necrosis-Factor plant, Behringwerke's Erythropoietin factory, and a Hoechst facility for insulin production, were all prevented from operating at various points in the late 1980s.[30]

Public opposition to biotechnology in Germany, however, did not completely stymie cancer research and testing using interleukins. Concerns about biotechnology became highly differentiated; German citizens worried about environmental impacts of modified microorganisms and feared harm to humans from DNA manipulation, but hoped for new therapeutics to treat life-threatening diseases. German physicians followed developments in the United States with great interest, and regular reports in journals such as the *Deutsches Ärzteblatt* kept the broader medical profession informed of progress with the interleukins and other new anticancer agents. Reports in the mid-1980s focused primarily on the outcomes of animal tests and early clinical trials. They also discussed the influence of private commercial interests and intense media publicity on clinical studies, including those run by the NCI.[31] Within a few years of the first tests in North America, German physicians also began experiments with "natural" IL-2. Rather than use the treatment on terminal cancer patients, however, initial clinical tests sought to immunize dialysis patients against hepatitis-B infection. Physicians at the Heidelberg Cancer Research Center thus hoped to first strengthen patients' immune systems before directly treating cancers.[32]

Proleukin in Germany

Cetus's newly formed European branch, Eurocetus, began clinical tests of IL-2 in 1986. Eurocetus trials eventually drew together data on 3,000 patients from Western and Central Europe, Russia, Hungary, and Israel. Unlike studies carried out in the United States, these tests sought to develop a dosage regimen not necessitating treatment in an intensive care unit. European physicians soon hit upon subcutaneous application as an alternative to the intravenous infusion used in the United States.[33] This approach reduced Proleukin's toxicity, since the compound was absorbed into the body more slowly than after intravenous injection. Significantly, it eliminated one of the main side effects of intravenous infusions. Capillary-leak syndrome had plagued Proleukin in the United States, but did not appear in the subcutaneous studies.[34] Furthermore, since this mode of administration was less invasive, patients could be treated in an ambulatory (outpatient) setting.

German and other European physicians also latched on to combination therapy of Proleukin with Interferon-alpha as helpful to outpatient or home care.[35] A series of reports in German medical journals suggested that subcutaneous infusion and combination therapy would result in fewer side effects, less strain on patients, and more successful treatment of cancer.[36] The approach drew sufficient interest from physicians that the company sponsored tests to document its efficacy and eventually presented data to the BGA supporting this method of application. Cetus used a database of 425 patients to compare 225 patients who received Proleukin as an intravenous drip infusion with 200 patients who injected themselves with Proleukin combined with Interferon-alpha. The two approaches did not result in statistically different outcomes in terms of cancer remission, but were strikingly different in their toxicity. Intravenous application had a remission rate of 15 percent, while 30 percent of the patients suffered from severe toxicity. In contrast, the subcutaneous application had a 20 percent remission rate with only 5 percent of patients experiencing severe toxicity.[37]

In the BGA application and in reports sent to German physicians, Eurocetus (absorbed into Chiron after its 1991 purchase of Cetus) explicitly criticized American treatment methods. In particular, side effects were seen as an outcome of the treatment method, not the treatment itself: "The treatment regimen developed by the NCI in Bethesda, Maryland, USA, is an intensive high-dose therapy protocol, which results in serious adverse reactions and in many cases, requires treatment in an intensive care unit. . . . Patient compliance can be greatly improved through the development of a less aggressive treatment regimen and better management of adverse reactions."[38]

Selection criteria for tests in Germany often excluded terminally ill patients, further reducing the frequency and severity of adverse reactions. Drawing on test results from the United States, German physicians avoided putting patients on Proleukin therapy who were likely to require intensive care. Employing a scale similar to ECOG, physicians divided patients with metastatic kidney cancer into four risk groups. According to the German pharmaceutical industry trade group (Bundesverband der Pharmazeutischen Industrie), patients in higher risk groups had little to gain from Proleukin therapy.[39] The miracle drug status first accorded to IL-2 in the United States had by this time given way to a much more measured approach. German physicians accordingly were less concerned with saving terminal patients than with treating patients at earlier stages of cancer.

Despite the success with Proleukin in ambulatory settings, BGA officials who approved the therapy in 1989 recommended treating metastatic kidney carcinoma only in hospital oncology departments or clinics with intensive medical supervision. According to government reviewers, Proleukin's biochemical impact on patients fit the regulatory category "not generally known to medical science."[40] They were especially concerned that its impact on patients varied so widely. Physicians who reviewed clinical studies for the BGA noted that the therapy only helped 25 percent of kidney cancer patients, while even fewer—10 percent—had complete remission.[41] The BGA therefore required Eurocetus to file regular reports of patient "experiences" after Proleukin's marketing. Just as advisory committee members in the United States wanted the company to supply the FDA with reports of ongoing studies, the German BGA wanted more data and reports than were found in the initial marketing application.

Brochures distributed by Chiron to German physicians as well as patients with kidney cancer clearly specify instances in which Proleukin should be avoided and describe potential drug interactions. In order for physicians to gather postmarket data, patients are advised to take an active part in their treatment, specifically by informing their doctors if they experience adverse effects such as heart pain or breathing difficulties. The "patient package insert" specifies that people should avoid the therapy if they spend more than 50 percent of their time in bed, suffer from an infection, or if their liver, kidneys, or other organs do not function properly.[42] As part of the marketing approval, physicians have to measure white blood cell counts and platelets to further weed out patients who should not be on the therapy. These restrictions helped BGA officials justify Proleukin's rapid approval in Germany. They also helped physicians select a controlled and homogeneous patient population for therapy.

In Germany, the interleukins generally, and IL-2 specifically, were often cited as prime examples of biotechnology's promise and failings. Critics claimed the treatment was inadequately tested and that recombinant Proleukin needed greater study and broader "societal consensus" before admission to widespread use.[43] As a result, when Eurocetus sought to bring Proleukin to the German market, the manufacturer went to great lengths to document both the "natural" presence of IL-2 in the human body and the environmental safety of its production methods. The German product monograph reveals the company's desire to convince government officials, physicians, and patients that Proleukin posed no special risks. A bold sidebar states, "The biological activity corresponds to that of natural IL-2," while the main text provides a detailed explanation of the manufacturing process. The monograph even reproduces the Proleukin DNA sequence, a half-page of A, C, T, and G letters (short for the four nucleotide base pairs—adenine, cytosine, thymine, and guanine—that make up DNA) that few readers could decode in terms of the product's biological activity.

More generally, the company went to great lengths to document that "natural and recombinant IL-2 induce comparable biological effects. . . . Both forms possess the same spectrum of biological activity and effects."[44] Public concerns about the equivalence of "natural" and "recombinant" ultimately had little direct impact on Proleukin's regulatory approval. They did, however, influence physicians to exercise great caution with the treatment. German physicians employed strict criteria to select patients, advanced a treatment method that could bypass the life-threatening capillary leak syndrome, and observed patients very closely for adverse reactions.

Clinical Trials and Clinical Care in the 1980s

The clinical testing and regulatory review of Proleukin exemplify two significant differences in the health care systems of the United States and Germany. First, responsibility for patient monitoring and treatment—especially after Proleukin had gained provisional approval in both countries—lay with the manufacturer in the United States and with the medical profession in Germany. This is not to say that physicians in the United States were irrelevant to Chiron when the company monitored patients and carried out postmarket clinical trials. Nonetheless, in many cases American physicians were little more than instruments of a data collection and analysis regime imposed by the FDA. In Germany, the medical profession had greater authority to shape the treatment regimen, and individual physicians served as crucial nodes in the flow of information between patients and the company and even between the company and the state. Physicians thus not only recorded and responded to side effects, they also played a formal role in determining Proleukin's marketing status during meetings with government officials and company representatives.

Second, American physicians advocated a testing protocol and treatment method that required long hospitalization periods for intravenous administration. German patients, considered by physicians to be reliable participants and subject to observation and control outside the hospital, often received treatment on an ambulatory basis through subcutaneous application. These two methods of administering Proleukin and structuring both trials and therapy are revealing of broader differences in patient autonomy between Germany and the United States. German physicians, under pressure from health insurers to pay more attention to expenditures, shied away from the financial costs and loss of authority associated with treating patients in intensive care units. They were able instead to configure their own clinics or even outpatient settings to meet the demands of Proleukin therapy. Patients had the appearance of greater autonomy and ability to lead "normal" day-to-day lives while on Proleukin.

In the United States, on the other hand, treatment in intensive care units helped maintain control over unruly subjects and eliminated some of the uncertainties of insurance reimbursement and potential liability from adverse reactions. Patients had little control over either the treatment regimen or any other aspect of their daily lives while receiving Proleukin. In both countries, clinical trials—before and after Proleukin's market authorization—served as sites for data collection and patient care. Despite their loss of autonomy in the intensive care unit, patients with terminal diseases in the United States played a greater role in debates over access to the experimental treatment than their German counterparts, a contrast that gained additional saliency with the rise of HIV-AIDS.

A New Politics of Testing and Care

Clinical trials came under different degrees of political scrutiny in the United States and Germany during the 1980s and 1990s. Disputes in the United States centered on access to medicines during testing, inclusion of women and minorities in clinical trials, and the reporting of results to wider audiences both during and after testing. These concerns changed the American institutional setting for access to experimental medicines. They also introduced new tensions to the dual role of clinical trials in determining safety and efficacy while also distributing potentially life-saving therapies to patients.

In contrast, clinical trials did not become sites for debates about patient inclusion, demographic representation, or institutional transparency in Germany. Germany's therapeutic culture discouraged patient activism and maintained a stable political conception of the patient. Concerns about testing methodology and procedural aspects of the regulatory process were confined to a more secluded network of industry, government, and medical profession. Cancer and AIDS activists played little if any role in changing the drug approval process. Rather than bring patient identity politics to the fore, disease-based interest groups focused their attention on more traditional concerns of access to treatment through the social welfare system and ensuring reimbursement of expensive therapies from financially squeezed insurers. Clinical trials, removed from the stage of public policy, remained a comparatively closed regime in which elite physicians assessed drug safety and efficacy. They were not a gateway to access medical care as in the United States.

Protest and Accommodation in the United States

AIDS activists in the United States not only protested slow drug approvals, but also criticized the structural constraints of clinical trials.[45] They brought public scrutiny and wider input to arguments about the number of participants necessary to prove drug safety and efficacy, access to data, how active a role patients could play, and, more broadly, the extent to which clinical trials should match complex, often contradictory, real world conditions. FDA regulations that specified methods for clinical trials and required each new drug application to include data from at least two controlled clinical trials led activists to target these issues as well. In particular, patient groups denounced screening methods, requirements for placebo use, and restrictions on trial participants. In editorials, speeches, protests, and direct correspondence with regulators, they argued for the inclusion of patients in various stages of the illness, and demanded the right to take other medicines during the course of a trial. Arguing that "real world" results would be more useful than clinical trials on ideal subjects, activists helped produce a shift to a more "pragmatic science" of drug testing.[46]

People with AIDS also challenged the authority of clinical trials and FDA oversight by carrying out underground tests of new drugs and threatening to sabotage NIH-sponsored trials through premature distribution of data or by ignoring trial protocols. For example, some participants in the 1986 trials of AZT also took dextran sulfate, imported from Japan through an underground "buyers' club." In other instances, underground tests, such as those carried out on the so-called "Compound Q," made drugs available to anyone who wanted them.[47] As AIDS patients became frustrated with the slow pace of formal trials, they organized community research initiatives to bring physicians and patients together. Routine interactions at a doctor's office now also served to collect data on experimental compounds.

Likewise, officially sanctioned trials underwent important changes as a large number of new compounds were tested in the late 1980s. Both AIDS and cancer patients considered participation in trials a means to obtain potentially life-saving drugs, rather than a voluntary contribution to the more abstract common good of furthering knowledge about experimental therapies. Adapting trial designs to acknowledge this perspective required broadening entry criteria and loosening requirements for controls.

With support of NIH officials and respected physicians sympathetic to the

AIDS movement, the FDA announced changes to its requirements for clinical trials in 1988. Previously, phase III testing had required the administration of experimental drugs and placebos—or other known treatments—to large patient populations in a double-blind, controlled clinical setting. Redesigning clinical trials to be more responsive to activists' suggestions, the FDA accepted historical controls rather than deny some sick patients access to a potentially useful medicine.[48] Further changes in clinical trial design were promoted by the AIDS Clinical Trials Group, which brought together patients, activists, clinical investigators, and government officials starting in 1989. Funded by the National Institute of Allergy and Infectious Diseases, the group advised physicians designing new drug trials to broaden entry criteria and to keep "patients and their advocates informed of interim findings."[49]

As described in Chapter 2, one response to the AIDS crisis in the United States was to speed drugs to market through a "parallel track" designated for promising treatments. After 1990, FDA officials could also allow new drugs on the market prior to the final compilation of safety and efficacy data. One track of the program maintained clinical trials as a carefully defined testing site, while the other enabled physicians to "provide drugs that had passed the Phase I test of safety to patients who were unable or unwilling to participate in regular clinical trials because they didn't meet the entry criteria for the standard trials, the trials were full, or they lived too far away from a trial site."[50]

In a further response to activists, the FDA began approving drugs based on surrogate endpoints, formalized in the 1992 "accelerated approval guidelines."[51] Rather than rely exclusively on measurable long-term survival, the FDA accepted changes in T-cell counts, measures of the amount of virus present in the blood, and other data as a surrogate for overall health. Regulatory review times declined rapidly in the early 1990s because of these changes.[52]

Noting the ability of AIDS activists to mobilize research funds and change the structure of drug trials, cancer patients and minority groups who had been either excluded from clinical testing or ignored by trial organizers also began pushing for greater access to experimental drugs and testing data. For example, the National Kidney Cancer Association (NKCA) formed in 1989 when patients met to discuss their experiences with kidney cancer and available treatment options. The original agenda of helping "patients obtain reimbursement for some experimental therapies" soon expanded to "empowering patients" to take an active role in treatment.[53] NKCA publications promote a shift in decision-making authority from the physician to the patient by reminding cancer patients that "your doctor works for you . . . you are his boss."[54] Cancer and AIDS activists thus paved the way for other organizations to represent patients and demand changes to the practice of medicine in the United States.

Following the 1993 establishment of an FDA Cancer Liaison Program to improve communication among FDA officials, cancer organizations, and patients, NKCA developed specific strategies for patients to gain access to experimental drugs. In booklets and brochures the organization described "Special Protocol Exceptions" and "Single Patient Investigational New Drug (IND) Applications" as means by which patients could get drugs even if they were not eligible for a specific trial. Under the protocol exemptions, local physicians can treat patients using procedures mapped out by the pharmaceutical company in its IND application. Physicians around the country can by this process take on the responsibilities of clinical investigators. The single patient IND can be used when a company has started clinical testing, but no clinical trial is underway for a specific type of cancer. This allows for individual treatment and care using otherwise unapproved medicines, but only under close physician supervision.

At the same time, more loosely designed clinical trials expanded to national and international scope. In effect, the transition from laboratory to the real world, long mediated by clinical trials, was now assisted by a broader concept of what constitutes a "clinic." Rather than only regulate pharmaceuticals at the point of market entry, FDA officials now sought to review information gathered along the entire spectrum from laboratory to final market approval.

Expanded access to new drugs and greater patient involvement in the regulatory process were further supported by several initiatives of the mid-1990s, including a National Performance Review that suggested ways to "reinvent the regulation of cancer drugs." Prompted by the executive branch's desire to accelerate drug approvals—particularly in the face of Republican threats to dismantle the FDA—the agency started accepting surrogate endpoints for cancer treatments in addition to AIDS therapies. In the past, tumor shrinkage had to be linked to "increased patient survival, decreased recurrence rate, increased disease-free interval, and / or improved quality of life" in order to count as evidence of drug efficacy.[55] Under the new approach, FDA medical officers accept partial tumor shrinkage as the principal measure of performance. Consequently, advisory committees began making recommendations for further research even as they voted to recommend FDA approval for drugs such as Proleukin.

A Changing Therapeutic Culture

Changes to the definition of "the clinic" promoted greater integration of testing and care. In this aspect, the American therapeutic culture began to look more like Germany's. Activists' criticisms, initially levied from an outsider stance, gradually changed to cooperation with the FDA and physicians directing clinical trials. Organizations that represented patients with AIDS, kidney cancer, and other diseases adopted greater restraint as they forged closer relationships with the medical establishment. By working with regulatory bodies and the medical community, activists earned recognition as "patient advocates" and received invitations to conferences and regulatory hearings on a regular basis. Larry Kramer, an outspoken AIDS activist and founder of ACT UP, worried about the resulting changes in activists' agenda: "When we were on the outside, fighting to get in, it was easier to call everyone names. But they were smart. They invited us inside. And we saw they looked human. And that makes hate harder."[56]

As characterized by Steven Epstein, the "professionalization of treatment activism," most notably among members of the Treatment Action Group (TAG), drew AIDS patients away from alternative therapies and led to splits within the activist community.[57] TAG drew the ire of other AIDS activists in 1994 when members concerned with the effectiveness of new HIV therapies urged the FDA to delay approval of Hoffman-LaRoche's application for saquinavir. Invoking more traditional standards for clinical trials, the group called for a long-term test with 18,000 subjects in order to ensure sufficient data on safety and efficacy. In the words of one analyst, "TAG broke away not only from virtually all other treatment activists in the country, but from the FDA itself."[58]

Nevertheless, FDA officials, drug company representatives, AIDS researchers, and representatives from activist organizations for the most part worked together in increasingly cordial arrangements by the mid-1990s. Just as the clinical trial had been broadened to incorporate outside perspectives, activists now wanted to ensure its survival as a scientific method. For example, during a 1995 NIH workshop on "Current Issues in AIDS Clinical Trials," David Barr of the Gay Men's Health Crisis argued in favor of premarket testing: "AIDS activists brag about how they cheat to get into a clinical trial. That is incredibly unethical. . . . We have to educate people about the value of AIDS research for ourselves and for those who follow."[59]

In order to encourage participants to stay in clinical trials rather than drop out to try other drugs or design their own drug regimen, workshop participants recommended allowing patients to enroll in more than one clinical trial, individualizing therapy according to patient progress rather than adhering to a strict timetable, and not insisting on the use of control drugs such as AZT. Although only one of many such meetings, the NIH workshop illustrates the extent to which scientists and government officials had changed their expectations for clinical trials in order to accommodate people with AIDS. Cooperation among regulators, physicians, and patients centered on methods for carrying out clinical trials while still getting drugs to patients. Advocates, for their part, came to believe that without disciplined clinical trial participants, testing results would be ambiguous, misleading, or even harmful to broader patient populations.

Efforts to simultaneously institutionalize wider participation in clinical trials and give patients greater say in the assessment of disease and treatment are signs that doctors and regulators realized that patient perceptions, emotional responses, and preferences and values play a significant role in treatment. By collecting both qualitative and quantitative data, and by broadening participant pools, reformers hoped that clinical trials could do more than just test new drugs. Trials in the United States became a site for treating disease, improving access to drugs, improving public participation in medical research, and changing testing procedures. Significantly, experimentation with new drugs became the locus for political negotiations among the four major actors in medical policy over access to medicines, representation, and the authority to speak for "the patient."

Forging Consensus in Germany

Beginning in the early 1980s, German AIDS patients and gay activists formed lobby groups and organizations to assist people with the disease. Even though far fewer HIV cases were recorded in Germany than in the United States (Figure 3), the spread of this untreatable disease similarly undermined assumptions about the infallibility of modern medical care. The founding of a national AIDS advisory council (AIDS-Beirat) in the mid-1980s consolidated smaller community-based organizations and provided additional funds for patient care and disease prevention efforts.[60] Chapter 2 mentioned the modest impact this organization and the Deutsche AIDS-Hilfe had on government legislation and drug regulation. The AIDS-Beirat sought to ease restrictions on clinical trials in the early 1990s, but concerns about access to medicines and criticisms of state and medical profession paternalism did not take center stage in Germany.

Patients and activists generally agreed with government officials that the 1976 Drug Law already accounted for contingencies associated with the emergence of a new and deadly disease. Responding to policy changes in the United States, the BGA in 1991 issued "official recommendations" concerning the pharmacological and toxicological tests it required prior to initiating clinical trials for AIDS drugs.[61] Government officials advised scientists to avoid duplicate pharmacology tests and reduce the time spent determining toxicity in animals. Official pronouncements of this type indicate how discussion of AIDS and access to medicines was framed in terms of technical details relating to drug testing. Access to test results, however, remained limited to the drug company, physicians conducting clinical trials, and government officials. Drug testing did not become a site for debates about representation or access to medicines, reinforcing traditional boundaries between experts and patients.

Further reinforcing traditional divisions in authority among physicians, patients, and the state, the German AIDS-Beirat opposed the introduction of HIV diagnostic tests that patients could perform on themselves. In a strongly worded press statement issued in July 1996, the AIDS-Beirat warned that only doctors and experienced laboratory personnel could accurately diagnose HIV. The organization suggested that patients rely on experts, rather than determine their own disease status through self-diagnosis.

Reliance on physicians extended from diagnosis to most aspects of patient care after a positive test result: "Physician advice, control and aid in psychosocial dimensions must be present in early phases of HIV infection and must begin with the moment of diagnosis. Recognition of possible HIV infection is a heavy burden for patients. The separation of testing and counseling is therefore dangerous, particularly since medical and psychosocial advising and care provide critical support for individuals coming to grips with a positive HIV antibody test result."[62]

Unlike groups pushing for greater patient autonomy in the United States, the AIDS-Beirat felt that HIV-positive individuals were best served by professional care using existing means for diagnosis and treatment. German patients largely accepted approaches to treatment criticized as "paternalistic" in the United States. Hence, neither the state nor physician autonomy was significantly challenged by the spread of AIDS in Germany.

Transparency and Participation

Different degrees of exposure of decision makers to surveillance and observation led to contrasts in procedural aspects of drug regulation during the 1980s and 1990s. New cooperative agreements, not wholly unlike those seen in the German "triangle of state—medical system—gay movement" were built up among the FDA, physicians, and AIDS activists in America.[63] Unlike the approach followed in Germany, however, meetings among these groups in the United States were well publicized and politically transparent. This allowed emerging disease-based organizations to rapidly gain political access. In order to allow for outside observation and in an effort to build consensus for alternative designs of clinical trials, frequent conferences and well-publicized announcements of even preliminary findings became the norm. In Germany, on the other hand, close working arrangements among state-recognized interest groups led to an institutional setting marked by friendly exchanges and only minor adjustment to preexisting modes of testing and regulating drugs. Few demands for greater transparency or access to still-experimental drugs meant that established institutional actors maintained a status quo built around a system of shared decision making. With no obvious routes to political access, disease organizations focused on public health and patient care, not changes to clinical trials and drug regulation. Remarkably, this system proved stable even when challenged by the apparently incurable AIDS epidemic.

Case 5. Indinavir: A Perfect Test?

The spread of HIV starting in the early 1980s and the emergence of AIDS activists in the mid-1980s posed a remarkable set of challenges to drug companies and government regulatory bodies. At first considered a form of cancer, the disease's means of transmission and etiology took years to resolve, making successful medical interventions difficult to design. While now accepted by nearly all scientists and medical authorities in the United States and Europe, the consensus that the retrovirus HIV causes the disease AIDS was challenged as recently as spring 2000 by South Africa's president, Thado Mbeki.[64] Controversy over AIDS causation stems partly from the extremely high price of available therapies, making alternative explanations for the disease and locally derived treatments appealing to poorer countries. Disputes over the source of AIDS, however, also reflect the failure of scientific medicine to find a cure for the disease.

Lingering questions about the root cause of AIDS have had little impact on research agendas at multinational pharmaceutical companies. In cooperation with government scientists and academic researchers, industry scientists have sought to kill the virus directly, interfere with HIV's ability to reproduce in the body, or confer immunity through a vaccine. The second of these three areas has proved most productive in terms of putting new drugs on the market. Starting in 1987, patients in the United States, Germany, and elsewhere could take the nucleoside analog AZT (Zidovudine) as a means to block reverse transcriptase, one of several enzymes necessary to viral reproduction in the body. Four years later, Merck scientists synthesized a compound that inhibits protease, an enzyme crucial to the replication of HIV. The company moved quickly to clinical studies once initial laboratory tests on indinavir, later marketed globally under the brand name Crixivan, showed promising results. After several years of small-scale safety tests and modifications to the dosage, Merck in 1994 initiated larger-scale clinical trials.[65]

These trials illustrate tensions between an emerging global testing and treatment regime on the one hand, and maintenance of national and regional regulatory styles on the other. The FDA and the European Agency for the Evaluation of Medicinal Products (EMEA), which largely superseded BGA authority for new drug applications by the mid-1990s, both approved the drug quickly. Nevertheless, important differences can be found between the United States and Europe in clinical trial design, the role of expertise, and public access to data on experimental medicines.

Crixivan in the United States

Crixivan's clinical testing and approval in the United States illustrate the impact activists had on FDA policies and procedures. At the same time, more than just government policies had changed; AIDS trials were also instrumental in forging new arrangements among patients, physicians, and industry. Merck worked closely with patient groups from an early stage of clinical research to plan trial protocols for Crixivan. The company launched clinical testing in January 1995 with a large multicenter trial that eventually incorporated some 4,800 patients in eleven countries. Activists soon prodded Merck and the FDA to make Crixivan even more widely available. Since the compound was metabolized quickly, large amounts of the drug had to be manufactured on short notice. Nearly a kilogram was required per patient each year. According to the company, "Manufacturing enough for an extensive worldwide trial would require that Merck's large-scale operations plant in Rahway, NJ and other facilities be fully dedicated to Crixivan."[66] Giving additional amounts to patients not in the clinical trials seemed impossible. Crixivan's limited availability led AIDS Project Los Angeles to report that the underground price for Crixivan would likely exceed $10,000 per year.[67]

Merck met regularly with a community advisory board and devised a lottery to pick 1,000 patients for its "compassionate use" program. Patients failing to meet entry criteria for the clinical trials thus had an opportunity to get Crixivan starting in 1994. The company coordinated enrollment, with widespread advertising through AIDS organizations and newsletters. The lottery narrowed qualified applicants to patients with CD4 counts (white blood cells crucial to the immune system) of 50 or less.[68] Despite this restriction, more than 11,000 people signed up for the 1,000 slots, indicating how quickly information about the drug had spread, even early in its clinical testing. Unlike the formal trials that required participants to visit clinics frequently for blood tests and other procedures, the compassionate use program had a loose structure. Patients' primary care physicians received a "regulatory package," including a trial protocol and consent form. Participants then met with their doctors to discuss the therapy and provide blood samples for testing, rather than having to travel to other clinics and meet with unfamiliar physicians.

Patient groups also clamored for access to protease inhibitors from Hoffman-LaRoche (saquinavir) and Abbott (norvir), who faced similar supply difficulties. Though lotteries offered a peculiarly American concept of an equitable solution in the short run, some observers expressed concerns about this precedent for distributing medicines for AIDS and cancer patients.[69] Scarcity of protease inhibitors during clinical testing, difficulties in manufacturing, and the necessity for free-market solutions all gave early indications that these drugs would be extremely costly when approved for wide-scale marketing. Furthermore, the extensive publicity surrounding each development with protease inhibitors led TAG members to question the pressure building toward accelerated approvals. In their view, rapid approvals often led to the marketing of drugs with harmful side effects and few long-term benefits for patients.

Merck submitted its new drug application to the FDA in early 1996, little more than a year after the launch of phase-III clinical trials. FDA officials and members of the Antiviral Drugs Advisory Committee worked extremely rapidly to review Crixivan, and the agency eventually approved it in a record-setting forty-two days. In line with American policies regarding public access and transparency, meetings of the advisory committee were announced ahead of time and public comments were solicited to aid deliberations on Crixivan's safety and activity. Facilitating public participation, the committee announced its meeting at a Maryland Holiday Inn a month in advance.[70] Like other advisory committee meetings, this one took place close to—but not actually in—FDA headquarters. The meeting included 385 outside attendees, an unusually large number for an FDA advisory committee and evidence of AIDS patients' excitement about the new treatment.

Company representatives spoke first at the advisory committee meeting, describing Crixivan's laboratory testing and results from patients who had received it in Phase I, II, and III trials. Next, the FDA analyzed Merck's application, pointing out strengths and weaknesses in the study designs and statistical analyses. Third, representatives from Project Inform, ACT UP, and other organizations described their cooperation with Merck and personal experiences with Crixivan therapy. Finally, the committee spent several hours discussing the application before voting to support an accelerated approval.

Merck's presentation described results from 2,000 patients who received Crixivan for at least three months, and 250 patients who took the drug for over a year. In the larger Phase II and III studies, Crixivan was tested alone and in combination with AZT and Epivir (3TC), another nucleoside analog.[71] Company officials presented data from the studies in a clear and consistent manner, going so far as to scale laboratory data similarly on most of their graphs. This facilitated a discussion among the advisory committee members that jumped back and forth between different studies. After describing the study designs, Merck argued that Crixivan was safe and efficacious based on quantified measures of serum viral RNA. Employing surrogate markers, in this case the "viral load," the company demonstrated statistical significance when comparing patients treated with Crixivan or a combination therapy to patients treated with AZT alone. To back up these results, Merck also documented a rebound of CD4 cell counts in patients on Crixivan. The company argued that patients' immune systems would recover quickly once Crixivan had suppressed HIV.

To prove that these results would apply beyond the confines of clinical trials, Merck representatives stressed the inclusiveness of the patient populations in the trials. Together, these patients displayed a broad range of CD4 cell counts, took a variety of anti-retroviral drugs before Crixivan, and were assigned to different "arms" of the study to explore the efficacy of combination therapies. Furthermore, Merck tracked the use of concomitant medications to uncover drug interactions with medicines not specifically part of the trial. The company next addressed patient demographics, stating, "in our Phase II trials, we set out to enroll patients who really reflected the demographics of the HIV epidemic. And within that, we wanted to try to enroll a substantial number of women."[72] Ultimately, the studies failed to find any gender-based differences, but Merck nonetheless assured committee members that they had maintained constant gender proportions throughout the clinical testing period by enrolling additional men or women when necessary. In this manner, Merck simultaneously responded to possible charges of gender inequality in its clinical trials and established that Crixivan had been tested in conditions analogous to those of patients taking multiple medications to fight AIDS.

Advisory committee members were clearly impressed by Merck's presentation but did turn the discussion more directly to Crixivan's side effects. The company acknowledged that some patients had developed a condition known as hyperbilirubinemia (an increase of bile in the bloodstream that can bring on jaundice), while others suffered from nephrolithiasis (kidney stones) during the clinical trials. Since less than 1 percent of patients experienced increased bilirubin levels, the company had not modified the protocol. The kidney stones, on the other hand, led clinicians to recommend that patients increase their fluid intake. Phase III studies showed a limited incidence of this side effect, indicating that greater consumption of water had helped mitigate formation of kidney stones.

FDA representatives at the meeting criticized the absence of some data from reports of two studies key to Merck's efficacy claims. Specifically, they noted that for three patients in study 028 (carried out in Brazil), the company had no CD4 cell counts once Crixivan therapy was started. For another six patients, Merck only reported partial data and failed to explain why these subjects had left the trial. Overall, the agency found that the company did not have full data on CD4 cell counts for 15 percent of the subjects in the two studies. Interestingly, the absence of complete CD4 cell count data did not invalidate the application in officials' minds. They were satisfied by Crixivan's ability to reduce the viral load and produce a durable response among patients. With three measures of efficacy available, FDA officials could be flexible about the precision and frequency of CD4 cell counts.

In public comments, patients and activists spoke directly about their strengthened immune systems, reduced viral loads, and new hope for survival despite the HIV infection. Their remarks intertwined touching personal narratives with quantitative measures of health and the biomedical discourse common to company and FDA presentations. For example, Linda Grinberg of the AIDS Research Alliance and Project Inform stated, "One year ago, with great effort, I dragged my sorry self before you, with 30 T4 cells . . . a soaring viral load, mounting health problems, and zero energy, begging for access to protease inhibitors. Today, I come before you, with renewed energy and almost 300 CD4 cells, to implore you, once again, to approve these drugs. My CD4 percentage has gone from 6 percent to as high as 22.4 percent. The Merck protease has given me back my life."[73]

Grinberg then sought to speed the decision-making process by describing the many "patients lying in hospital beds with IV tubes" while advisory committee members debated Crixivan's merits. Invoking a dichotomy between the real world of patient suffering and the sanitized world of committee meetings and medical discussion, she asked, "In our pursuit of better data, what are the sacrifices?" Speaking directly to the committee members and FDA representatives, Grinberg argued forcefully that patient care and a variety of therapeutic options—including Crixivan—were more important than perfect data sets or complete proof of efficacy.

Not all of the public commentary involved personal narratives or portrayals of suffering patients. For example, Spencer Cox from the Treatment Action Group raised concerns about Merck's application based on the company's failure to find the optimal point in a patient's disease history at which to initiate Crixivan therapy. Clinical trials had not resolved whether it was better to start therapy as soon as HIV was identified in a patient, or to wait until they exhibited symptoms of full-blown AIDS. He noted that it would be "unfair" to lay this solely on Merck, since the question applied equally to other therapies. Instead, he sought to sway committee members to pressure companies to design a separate set of trials regarding the optimal point to start therapy with protease inhibitors.[74] Finally, Jules Levin of the National AIDS Treatment Advocacy Project and Rob Camp from the European AIDS Treatment Group underscored the importance of committee members' votes for AIDS patients around the world. As Camp put it, "The whole world is watching these proceedings. We, even in Europe, live with the decisions and decision-making process that happens here."[75]

When responding to the company, the FDA, and patient representatives, advisory committee members focused on adverse reactions, adherence to the treatment regimen, and research that Merck should carry out after Crixivan's approval. Kidney stones were an obvious concern, and committee members asked about hospitalization rates and recovery among patients who discontinued therapy. Committee members also were curious about reactions to the combination therapy, requesting comparative data across the two- and three-drug treatments. Some of the results worried them, leading one member to ask the FDA if Merck would be required to compile additional reports and verify surrogate results once Crixivan had been in use for a longer time period.[76]

Noting that regular and frequent consumption of Crixivan was vital to its efficacy, committee members asked Merck how the company had ensured compliance during clinical trials and what it would do once the drug was marketed. Merck's representatives explained that patients in the trials filled out "diary cards" to record when they took their medicine. As a backup, study coordinators counted capsules in the patient's possession and discussed any discrepancies with them. While not keeping patients in intensive care units as in the Proleukin case, this approach disciplined patients to adhere to a strict protocol. Once the drug was on the market, Merck set up an interactive "livin' it" program of "colorful, easy-to-read materials, checklists and planning guides to help patients manage their therapy."[77] Patients who use a web-based "custom pill planner" can establish a daily routine with activities to remind them when it is "pill time."[78]

Finally, advisory committee members expressed their concerns, both specifically to Merck and more generally to FDA officials (including Commissioner David Kessler) that it would be difficult to carry out long-term clinical trials and compile valid endpoint data if Crixivan were marketed as an "accelerated approval." Noting that many AIDS patients would not be able to afford the drug, committee members suggested that Merck continue to recruit patients into long-term clinical studies. At the same time, they recognized that postmarket studies would likely attract only patients who lacked insurance and could not afford the drug on their own, further underscoring a "two-tier health care system" that forces poor people to serve as research subjects.[79]

The ethics of contributing to this feature of American health care clearly disturbed some members of the advisory committee. Merck responded that the company would "obtain as much information in terms of the long-term safety of the drug by continuing [to monitor] groups of patients for very long periods of time on therapy." The company also committed to carrying out "outcomes" studies—with protocols to be negotiated between the company and the FDA—to verify the early results. With these assurances, committee members voted in favor of the accelerated review and gave their formal support to the multi-drug combination therapy.

Crixivan was approved both as an independent therapy and for use in combination with nucleoside analogs such as AZT two weeks later. The accelerated approval was based on official review of two controlled clinical trials involving 490 patients and a small study on patients taking Crixivan in combination with both AZT and Epivir. As the FDA reported in a press release, these trials divided patients into three groups. One group received Crixivan alone, another took the drug in combination with AZT, and a third was treated with just AZT.[80] From 2,000 patients described in the advisory committee meeting, Merck limited its final application to the FDA to fewer than 500 patients. Agreeing with the company, FDA officials accepted the surrogate markers of viral load and CD4 cell counts as evidence of Crixivan's efficacy.

In the immediate aftermath of Crixivan's approval, its availability again took center stage. Since Merck only had limited supplies available, it was forced to ration the drug for the first several months. Not surprisingly, this dominated discussions among activist groups, especially when Merck chose a mail-order pharmacy, Stadtlanders, as the sole distributor. In response to criticism, Merck officials explained that antitrust laws prevented them from negotiating a fixed price with Stadtlanders or pressuring the distributor to lower its market price, set at $5,280 per year, a 32 percent markup over Merck's price. As one commentator probed, "Is it OK for Stadtlanders to be given an absolute monopoly of a life-critical drug, be allowed to set whatever price it wants, and then use this situation to set an unusually high markup? Is it OK for Merck to wash its hands in the antitrust laws?"[81]

Merck eventually resolved the issue by building new factories to increase production and made Crixivan available through competing distributors. Price concerns, however, did not completely go away. Earlier comments made by FDA advisory committee members regarding the expense of treating patients with multiple drugs proved unfortunately prescient.

The shift in the United States to rapid marketing authorization has been accompanied by the requirement to study drugs long after the initial approval. Companies such as Merck get accelerated approval for drugs with the understanding that they will monitor patients and carefully document side effects for years to come. As a result of reports filed with the agency, the FDA began warning physicians and patients in June 1997 that protease inhibitors can raise blood sugar levels and even can cause diabetes. In public announcements, FDA officials described 83 cases of new or exacerbated diabetes mellitus and hyperglycemia. In response, an FDA bulletin sent to physicians and patients stated, "Based on present information, FDA believes that the benefits of these drugs to patients suffering from HIV infection outweigh the various risks of taking the drugs."[82] Patients, the agency recognized, could control diabetes using other treatments, including insulin therapy. AIDS, on the other hand, could only be treated effectively using the multi-drug therapy of protease inhibitors and nucleoside analogs. By the late 1990s, then, the FDA had not only sped up its drug approval practices, but had also modified risk calculations to give the benefit of the doubt to patients desiring access to drugs, rather than cutting off access to a therapy because of side effects.

Crixivan in a "Harmonized" Europe

Merck's United Kingdom division submitted an application to EMEA in March 1996, almost simultaneously with the U.S. application. While much of the application is unavailable to the public, the European Public Assessment Report (EPAR) offers a detailed description of steps taken in the assessment of Crixivan. First, several "rapporteurs" were assigned to oversee the application and review Crixivan's safety and efficacy. Next, a board known as the Commission on Proprietary Medicinal Products (CPMP) examined this report along with the original application. Assessment teams grouped by their expertise in toxicology, pharmacology, and clinical trials then prepared questions for the company, which the CPMP sent to Merck at the end of May. The company responded nine days later and also met with reviewers in mid-June to discuss ongoing clinical studies. Reflecting the closed character of European expert proceedings, the EPAR provides no additional details on the content of questions posed to the company or the nature of interactions between Merck and CPMP reviewers. CPMP members soon issued a positive opinion of the application and the European Commission officially approved the drug in early October. The review period was longer than in the United States, but still met official guidelines of 210 days or less. Meetings were not publicly announced at any point in this process, nor were opportunities given for commentary from patients or physicians not officially responsible for reviewing the application.

Crixivan's approval report begins with an abstract of the marketing authorization for its use to treat HIV in combination with anti-retroviral drugs. Adopting the same surrogate markers to gauge Crixivan's efficacy as were used in the United States, reviewers wrote, "The combination of Indinavir with zidovudine (AZT) / didanosine (ddI) . . . reduced the amount of human immunodeficiency virus in serum and increases CD4 cell counts."[83] This medical finding allowed EMEA to approve Crixivan, even though reviewers suggested that, since efficacy was based on biological markers and clinical endpoints, "the marketing authorization holder is *requested* to submit results of ongoing clinical studies."[84] The EPAR then moves rapidly to technical details of Crixivan's composition, stability, pharmacodynamics, toxicology, and pharmacokinetics.

Clinical trials of Crixivan were presented in tabular form in the public assessment report. As underscored by BUKO-Pharmakampagne, a German group critical of pharmaceutical industry practices, the format offers few useful details for patients curious about treatment options.[85] The EPAR presented

Phase II trials, termed "dose finding studies," in a table listing the length of the study period and the number of subjects. Results of the Crixivan trials were compared to other treatments, especially AZT when taken alone. Phase III trials, generally considered key to determining efficacy, are described as "confirmatory trials," since Crixivan's early success had put it on an accelerated track.

Accelerated review in the EU mimics the FDA's approach to speeding approvals for life-threatening illnesses. The EPAR report, however, provides little data on people who took Crixivan or about their experiences with the drug. It does state that 417 patients enrolled in eight phase II trials, and that Merck conducted five large-scale phase III trials. Only seven of these fifteen studies are described in any detail. In contrast to developments in the United States, specifics of the studies and their design were not a topic of open debate in Europe. As a result, there was less discussion about additional clinical research or procedures for maintaining patient compliance with the therapy in Europe than in the United States. Instead, as was the case for Germany, the European therapeutic culture allowed physicians and other medical experts to speak for the patient in regulatory decisions.

European Regulatory Culture

EMEA began reviewing drug applications in January 1996, making Crixivan one of the first products approved by this new pan-European regulatory agency. The harmonized central review process explicitly seeks to promote Europe as a site for clinical research and investment by multinational pharmaceutical firms.[86] EMEA's mission statement thus advances "timely access" to "innovative medicines," and annual reports stress that the "mean processing time" for new drug applications is well below a 240-day target.[87] EMEA reports to the E.U. Directorate-General for Industry, specifically the Unit for Pharmaceuticals and Cosmetics (DG III / E / 3), though the agency also maintain contacts with the Directorate for Consumer Policy and Consumer Health Protection. Its ability to review applications quickly stems at least partly from close collaboration among medical experts, representatives from national regulatory agencies, and drug company scientists in the centralized review process. In effect, EMEA has adopted a regulatory approach whereby selected experts make decisions in closed meetings.[88] Consensus politics dominate decision making, not least because the rapporteur in charge of the review is suggested by the company and, in turn, chooses experts for the CPMP panel. Furthermore, CPMP decisions are not subject to challenge by national regulatory authorities, interested medical professionals, or patients in E.U. countries.

Indicative less of direct outside agitation than of an effort to build a constituency among pharmaceutical companies and the medical profession, EMEA promotes transparency and access to documents as interrelated governing approaches. Transparency is intended to strengthen "the democratic nature of the institutions and the public's confidence in the administration."[89] As implemented by EMEA, however, transparency largely means access to a limited set of documents on the Internet, including annual reports, press releases, meeting calendars, and EMEA's official policies. Policies for transparency and document access are readily available, whereas detailed information about approved drugs or medicines under review are more difficult to obtain.

For patients, physicians, or others interested in more detailed materials, EMEA has created a "freedom of information" mechanism whereby they can request documents.[90] Access to materials, however, is carefully orchestrated and tightly controlled by agency officials. Documents not available to the public include draft statements, agendas or minutes of meetings, materials relating to the preparation of scientific opinions, correspondence between experts or with applicant companies, and items including companies' proprietary knowledge. Of the material made available, the EPARs have been the most popular, with an average of 15,000 copies requested for each approved drug.

Materials included in an EPAR are screened for proprietary data, specifics about clinical trial participants, or information that in experts' assessments might mislead patients. Reports therefore offer very general data about a new drug. Noting this, some critics have accused the agency of failing to link transparency to useful medical information: "Openness would permit consumers (both doctors and patients) greater understanding of the drugs available and offer a way of checking against potential abuse and incompetence of the regulatory authorities."[91]

Similar to developments in the United States, these critics want the public to oversee and influence regulatory decision making. This push for an individualization of oversight and greater access to the government is a comparatively recent development in Europe, where, as we have seen, the terrain of drug regulation was historically divided among states, the medical profession, and industry. Materials made available under EMEA transparency guidelines are a move toward facilitating greater review and observation of the agency by individual patients and physicians. Nevertheless, concerns about demographic representation in clinical trials and greater access to scientific and medical information about marketed drugs are only now starting to influence regulatory policy.

While EMEA is pursuing transparency, it maintains a state-centered system of data collection and review. The Crixivan EPAR illustrates that patients seeking to find out what other people experienced during the course of clinical trials can only uncover summary data on viral loads and CD4 cell counts. In order to make further decisions regarding treatment, they must work within the existing network of regulatory bodies, the pharmaceutical industry, and medical associations. This does not mean that a given treatment will be any less efficacious than in the more transparent United States. Patients in Europe, however, must develop long-standing relationships of trust with their physicians in order to have access to medical information more publicly available in America.

Knowing Subjects

Taken together, the case studies of Proleukin and Crixivan illustrate important changes to drug testing in the last two decades. Patients with cancer and AIDS in the United States attacked FDA risk assessment policies and demanded the right to individually assume risks associated with imperfectly tested drugs. They also drew attention to a "scientific bias" in clinical trials that inhibited the production of real world knowledge about new medicines. Public engagement with clinical trials had significant impact on the construction of risk profiles by the FDA and its advisory committees. Instead of limiting their focus to trade-offs between safety and adverse reactions, they now openly accepted a language of "access to drugs" and the "right to obtain treatment." In Germany, on the other hand, criticism was levied against clinical studies of drugs "looking for diseases." Human experiments using interleukins and other biotechnology-based medicines were considered unethical, especially when efforts were made to try out an array of compounds on dying patients. Rather than considering drug tests a means to access possible cures, critics decried them for trying out powerful drugs on the country's weakest, most diseased citizens.

Clinical trials grew in significance between 1980 and 2000 as a technology for resolving both medical questions about drug safety and efficacy as well as political concerns about representation in the United States and harmonization in Europe. The clinical trial now more than ever before involved government actors, disease-based organizations, and doctors and patients interacting outside the traditional doctor-patient relationship. Responding to activists in the United States, drug testing changed from a strict input-output system to appear something more like the German approach combining care and testing. Unlike in Germany, however, clinical trials also were called upon to negotiate broader questions of political representation and access to decision making. Changes were underway in Germany as well, once implementation of the 1976 drug law set restrictions on who could direct clinical trials and increased the role of government regulators to review results. With expansion of EU regulatory authority, trials now also served as public displays of pan-European governance.

Harmonized procedures for drug approval across Europe incorporate public transparency—long a hallmark of the American political system—to help legitimate and attract public support for EMEA. Yet the kinds of transparency and access found in Europe and the United States remain fundamentally different. Even though Proleukin and Crixivan were approved in both regions, the climates for testing, regulatory review, and manufacturing display striking contrasts in political mobilization and institutional responses. While environmental groups in Germany called for greater regulatory control over biotechnology and mobilized to prevent the manufacture of medicines through genetic engineering, disease-based activists in the United States pressed for fewer regulations, less premarket testing, and immediate access to drugs. In the absence of national health insurance in the United States—or even a coordinated private system as found in Germany—unmet social and medical needs found expression in political mobilization.

The contrast between environmental activists pushing for more regulation in one country and patient activists demanding less intrusive government oversight in the other is revealing about the underlying therapeutic cultures in the United States and Germany. American AIDS and cancer activists offer a remarkable success story of increased access to information and in their ability to redefine "the patient" in political discourse and regulatory policy. They also demonstrated the ability of lay experts to educate themselves about technical procedures and articulate their positions in a persuasive manner. In a country offering little in the way of comprehensive insurance or government assurance of long-term care, patients opened clinical trials to greater scrutiny and used them to get medical treatment. Germany has seen little mobilization around specific diseases; instead the very necessity of additional expensive therapeutics at least briefly came under challenge. A lack of trust in expert assessments of risks from biotechnology has spilled over to the drug review and approval process as well. Consequently, the German public increasingly asks for greater precautionary regulation and additional premarket testing of medicines.

Initiatives in the United States to expand access to experimental drugs and approve medicines using surrogate endpoints rely on the observation of patients even after drugs are widely marketed. In effect, the older approach of extensive premarket testing and comparatively slow review by government officials was traded for a still poorly defined system in which patients participate in long-term surveillance as they take prescription drugs. Historically a success in Germany, this approach may transfer poorly to diseases other than cancer and AIDS. Patients with life-threatening conditions are understandably motivated to interact with long-term research outside the tightly controlled clinical domain. Yet while barriers between the clinic and market have been relaxed in the United States, little has been done to make physicians more accessible to those experiencing adverse reactions. Coupled to a broader concept of "the clinic," physicians are now asked to monitor patients for years or even decades. The immense scope of this surveillance means that long periods may pass between moments of data collection that offer opportunities for individual patient care. As the next chapter describes, systems for collecting and standardizing reports of adverse reactions differ between the two countries, paralleling the contrast in the premarket domain between state centralization in the United States and greater diffusion of responsibility among the medical profession, industry, and the government in Germany.

5

Configuring the Market as a Testing Site

DESPITE EFFORTS TO TEST MEDICINES BEFORE THEY come into widespread use, adverse reactions and undesired side effects (*unerwünschte Nebenwirkungen*) often plague marketed drugs. Over the course of the last fifty years, centralized systems were established in both the United States and Germany to monitor side effects and collect reports about drugs. Postmarketing surveillance, often termed pharmacovigilance, extended the boundaries of testing beyond clinical trials into routine drug therapy. As in clinical testing, methods used to collect and standardize reports of adverse reactions reflect national differences in the social roles and political authority of physicians, industry, and the government. Contrasts between the American and German therapeutic cultures shaped the institutional terrain for collecting and responding to reports of side effects, and approaches followed to create databases about marketed drugs. Specifically, they contributed to a push for quantifiable data in the United States and promoted qualitative review of side effects in Germany.

Just as in legislative debates about drug laws and disputes over the design of clinical trials, a series of negotiations concerning the social roles and political standing of "the patient" were crucial to the evolution of pharmacovigilance. Organizations that identified and responded to adverse reactions in the United States and Germany had to mediate among competing visions of patients presented by physicians, industry, the state, and disease-based interest groups. These same organizations were then confronted by the reality of physicians unwilling or, at a minimum, reluctant to record and share intimate details of their patients' experiences with drugs. Norms for patient care, medical observation, and privacy shaped what kinds of information were collected and how it could be standardized and compared. These normative aspects of American and German therapeutic cultures strongly influenced institutional responses to adverse reactions, much as in premarket testing.

Pharmacovigilance joins with legal / regulatory codes and clinical testing as a third key element of each country's unique therapeutic culture. This chapter pays close attention to differences between institutional frameworks that compile reports of side effects and decide when a drug should be removed from the market. In the United States, the American Medical Association's (AMA) Council on Drugs collected reports of side effects and put pressure on drug manufacturers to withdraw dangerous drugs between the mid-1950s and late 1960s. At that point, the Food and Drug Administration (FDA) created a centralized system for data collection and review. The agency also set formal guidelines for drug performance and forced companies to withdraw unsafe or ineffective medicines.

In Germany, on the other hand, the Federal Chamber of Physicians' Drug Commission (Arzneimittelkommission der deutschen Ärzteschaft, or AkdÄ) was the only organization to collect and respond to reports of adverse reactions during the first third of the century. This professional association reasserted its position after the Second World War and maintained its status to the present by helping to design a formal system for risk assessment and response known as the "step-plan" (*Stufenplan*). While the Federal Institute for Pharmaceutical and Medicinal Products (Bundesinstitut für Arzneimittel- und Medizinprodukte, or BfArM) now serves as the central regulatory authority, AkdÄ retains an important voice in decisions on drug withdrawals. Differences between these two systems illustrate not only shifts in expert authority and autonomy over time in each country, but also further document important national contrasts in the construction of the patient for purposes of drug regulation.

Testing from Clinic to Market

Prescription drugs are taken by ethnically diverse patients who live in a variety of geographic areas, face disparate economic circumstances, consume a range of diets, and often follow daily routines nothing like those of subjects who participated in clinical trials. Substantial efforts are required to oversee the enormous variability found among patients and treatment settings once drugs are on the market. Organizations involved in pharmacovigilance have to seek out patient populations at risk from approved drugs. In contrast to the more selective process of choosing individuals for participation in clinical trials, postmarket oversight potentially must observe every patient ↔ drug interaction in order to gather convincing evidence.

Trying to make this vast terrain manageable, medical associations in the United States and Germany established commissions and committees to collect reports on marketed drugs by the middle of the twentieth century. These professional groups sought to assert control over the drug market in both countries by carrying out additional drug tests, controlling advertising in key journals, and publicizing instances of adverse drug reactions. Physicians in this manner shifted the locus for data collection from the narrow confines of the clinical trial to society at large.

At the same time, organizations in both countries restructured everyday doctor-patient interactions to serve as clinical trial surrogates. They tried to gather enough information to document adverse reactions without incorporating so many variables as to preclude meaningful causal connections. "Raising the world" from a "laboratory," as Bruno Latour has noted, involves a double movement of laboratory to the field and field to the laboratory.[1] In the case of pharmacovigilance, data collection shifted from the clinical trial to the market; at the same time, the market was forcibly reconfigured as an extension of the clinical trial. Just as clinical trials gradually moved out of lab-like settings, so therapy in a physician's office or at a patient's home became part of a drug's field study.

Physicians collecting reports on marketed drugs face a quandary regarding the projection from "test to actual use of the *user*."[2] Tests, especially clinical trials, tend to incorporate a narrow population of subjects. Once a drug is approved, however, companies want to promote its use among a broader spectrum of patients. They also lobby physicians to prescribe it for a variety of medical conditions. Organizations that collected reports of side effects in both the United States and Germany warned physicians that many of these uses were never actually tested in the clinical trial.

Building a bridge between clinical trials and adverse reaction reporting, they tried to convince practicing physicians that side effects relate to a manageable number of variables. They advocated seeing drug therapy in terms of data sets limited to patient age, weight, race, and a small number of other features in order to abstract and standardize the complexities of medical care. Mild reactions such as skin rashes, dizziness, and difficulty breathing, as well as serious events including birth defects and death, are abstracted from the individual patient to medical case reports. In turn, reports can be compared with one another after the "adverse events" are categorized according to a standard list of reactions. Ideally, this process narrows the spectrum of potential links between drugs and an outbreak of adverse reactions. In practice, physicians find it difficult to narrow the diversity of patients' experiences with drugs to fit categories on standardized reporting forms.

The construction of causal relationships between pharmaceuticals and side effects depends on several translations integral to postmarketing review mechanisms. First, a patient's self-analysis is converted to the professional language of physicians. Reports of discomfort or serious adverse outcomes are written up into professional case reports. Next, drug firms, medical associations, and regulatory agencies compile reports in order to produce aggregate data and statistical evaluations. Standardized reporting forms and formal agreements among physicians, industry, and the government mediate these two translations; first from patient description to medical diagnosis, then from case report to statistical table. Throughout, the process matches the "translation exercises" that sociologists of science have identified as a crucial element of generating and confirming scientific evidence.[3] Intriguingly, government agencies and professional societies followed different methods for these translations in the United States and Germany. In the United States, the FDA sought to quantify adverse reactions, whereas in Germany, the medical association based decisions on the professional expertise of practicing doctors.

Medical associations in both countries initiated efforts to gather and compare complaints about drugs. Noting the excessive optimism surrounding antibiotics in the 1950s, they sought to inform practicing doctors of the dangers associated with this "golden age" of drug therapy. Associations also tried to recruit and train members to serve as data collectors. In the United States, however, the AMA failed to attract widespread participation and lacked the resources needed to standardize disparate reports from doctor's offices, small medical clinics, and large hospitals. When the FDA began carrying out detailed postmarket studies at research hospitals, the AMA stopped its efforts. Physicians in the United States now report cases of side effects either to the manufacturer, the FDA, or both. In Germany, AkdÄ was able to enroll physicians and maintained its medical and political status even when challenged by the federal government and the pharmaceutical industry. A network incorporating the medical profession, government, and drug industry now collects and shares reports of side effects.

These institutional differences arose from a sharp divergence in how the patient was conceptualized and even operationalized as an actor in the two countries. In the United States, attention shifted from individual case reports to group and population studies. Translating local reports into aggregate data sets was part of an effort to bypass the local expertise and supposedly biased assessments of practicing doctors. The FDA made this happen by converting individual case reports into large data sets for quantitative analysis. The government's vision of patients needing protection from industry drove this process. As part of the emergence of a free-market model for information flow, the FDA recently started to collect reports directly from patients, thereby circumventing physicians completely. In Germany, expert judgment was based on detailed information collected from smaller data sets. Linked to their authority over the clinic and ability to speak for the patient, physicians could more readily defend their professional expertise and control over the domain of side effects. Even though a broad network of organizations exchanges information about drugs, physicians filter reports before they become case data.

Postmarketing Oversight by the Medical Profession, 1950–1970

The Medical Profession in America

Responding to early-twentieth-century concerns about drug safety, the AMA launched a Council on Pharmacy and Chemistry in 1905.[4] Council members included pharmacologists, chemists, and physicians drawn from universities and government agencies. They published standards for drug quality and created a voluntary "Seal of Acceptance" program to evaluate drug safety and efficacy. When the council concluded that a given drug was unsafe, it blocked advertising in the *Journal of the American Medical Association* (*JAMA*).[5] Council members also published a list of drugs that met their laboratory and clinical standards: the *New and Nonofficial Remedies*.

JAMA's refusal to print advertisements for ineffective or impure drugs helped establish boundaries between "scientific" medicines and so-called "nostrums."[6] By demarcating good drugs from bad, council members influenced the prescribing practices of physicians around the country. Companies that bypassed council tests and ignored the Seal of Acceptance Program found it difficult to market their drugs to the mainstream medical profession.

In 1955, the council dropped its Seal of Acceptance Program and started building a registry of adverse reactions. This change resulted from a lack of funds to support the Seal Program as well as changes at the AMA and *JAMA*. The AMA's ability to control advertising in its journal had positioned the society as a gatekeeper of sorts between companies and physicians. During the first half of the century, the council could levy a quality and safety toll on producers. Once advertising revenue became a crucial source of funding for the AMA, drug companies gained financial leverage over *JAMA* editors and the council's regulatory authority. Council activities then came under fire as an unnecessary barrier to market entry.[7]

The reorganized Council on Drugs sought to position itself as a national monitor of patients' experiences with pharmaceuticals, rather than serving as a gatekeeper between industry and physicians. Severe side effects associated with the antibiotic chloramphenicol provided additional justification for this organizational change.[8] Between 1953 and 1955, reports in medical journals documented nearly 400 cases of aplastic anemia, an often fatal condition in which the bone marrow stops producing red or white blood cells.[9] The Council on Drugs quickly established a Committee on Blood Dyscrasias that eventually linked cases of aplastic anemia to chloramphenicol.

Following the committee's success in identifying chloramphenicol as the cause of aplastic anemia cases, its mandate was broadened in 1960 to include the review of all adverse drug reactions. Members of this expanded Committee on Adverse Reactions developed an official registry of side effects. Committee members hoped that physicians in private practice would report to their centralized site. Hospitals were expected to provide additional data. When the committee surveyed 986 hospitals in 1965, however, only 386 (39 percent) collected reports of adverse drug reactions and shared them with the AMA.[10] In a bid to expand the council's authority, its chairman, Harry Dowling, asked the Joint Commission on Accreditation of Hospitals to make reporting mandatory for new members. The Joint Commission declined Dowling's request.

Greater resources were brought to bear in efforts to recruit physicians as data collectors. A standardized form was published yearly in *JAMA* (Figure 4), and the committee sent additional copies directly to doctors.[11] Forms gathered information about a specific adverse reaction, the patient, and the physician. In particular, the committee was interested in learning a patient's occupation, age, weight, race, and sex. Doctors also were asked to provide a case history, information about their diagnostic approaches, and to list all prescription drugs and potentially toxic agents the patient had taken in the previous half year. Committee members then reviewed reports to find dangerous interactions among prescription drugs or to identify pharmaceuticals that caused specific side effects. Despite collecting demographic data, little effort was expended to connect adverse reactions with patients' professions, races, gender, weight, or age. Nevertheless, case histories, descriptions of diagnostic methods, and lists of prescribed drugs gave committee members a tool with which they could oversee medical care in the United States.

The AMA's staff compiled reports and then distributed them to committee panels organized around types of reactions and suspicious drugs. Comparing reports posed a significant challenge to the committee, even though the forms were structured to obtain information in a concise and standardized format.

For AMA use only	REGISTRY ON ADVERSE REACTIONS—COUNCIL ON DRUGS

AMERICAN MEDICAL ASSOCIATION, 535 North Dearborn Street, Chicago, Illinois 60610

See Guide For Reporting for special instructions and glossary to aid you in completing this form. If you wish to add any material, please enclose a separate sheet.

1. a. Patient's Initials____ ____ ____ b. Sex____ c. Weight____
d. Date of Birth_____ e. Occupation_____
   Mo./Day/Yr.
f. 1. ☐ Cauc. 2. ☐ Negro 3. ☐ Oriental
   4. ☐ Amer. Indian 5. ☐ Other

2. a. Dr._____
b. Street_____
   City_____ State_____ Zip Code____
c. Date_____

3. Adverse Reaction(s) (Describe)

4. a. Date of Onset_____ b. Date of Diagnosis_____ c. Was onset of reaction { 1. ☐ acute explosive / 2. ☐ slowly developing

5. a. Result of Relevant Diagnostic Studies (Clinical Laboratory, Endoscopy, Biopsy, Autopsy, X-Ray, etc.):

b. Pathologist_____ Hospital_____ Tissue available? yes ☐ no ☐

6. List all drugs patient has received in the 6 months prior to onset of adverse reaction. Include biologicals, diagnostic agents, and transfusions.

Give manufacturer's name and lot or code number, if available. Indicate date of first and last dose of drug for each course of therapy, and indicate route of administration.

NAME OF DRUG (Trade Name)	TOTAL DAILY DOSE	ROUTE (p.o., im, iv, etc.)	DURATION OF THERAPY (Days)	DATES OF ADMINISTRATION Date started Date ended	DISORDER OR REASON FOR USE OF DRUG
(suspected drug)					

7. List all potentially toxic agents to which patient has been exposed, and describe circumstances of exposure. Give any information available on dose or exposure. (Include radiation, household products, industrial and agricultural chemicals, cosmetics, etc.)

Name and Type of Agent	Type & Description of Exposure	Amount, Dosage and Duration

8. a. Has patient been exposed to suspected drug or agent before? ☐ Yes ☐ No

b. Was suspect drug or agent used according to directions? ☐ Yes ☐ No Explain_____

9. Other Disorders Which Existed Prior to Onset of Adverse Reaction or Are Now Present:

10. Factors Contributing to Reaction (check all applicable boxes):
a. 1 ☐ self medication by patient b. 1 ☐ drug mislabeled
2 ☐ accidental exposure   2 ☐ decomposition of drug
3 ☐ occupational exposure   3 ☐ contamination of drug
Comments: 4 ☐ drug outdated
   5 ☐ interaction of two or more drugs

11. Outcome of Case
1 ☐ Recovered   4 ☐ Died_____
2 ☐ Alive with sequelae
   (date and cause of death)
Explain_____
3 ☐ Still under Treatment 5 ☐ Autopsy (Describe in item 5)

12. Sources of Suspected Drug:
1 ☐ from physician   5 ☐ other retail source
2 ☐ physician's sample 6 ☐ mail order
3 ☐ hospital   7 ☐ door-to-door salesman
4 ☐ pharmacy

13. a. Has this case been reported to any other group or agency?
☐ FDA ☐ Mfr. ☐ Poison Control Center ☐ Other (specify)
b. Has or will this case appear in the literature?
☐ Yes ☐ No Journal Ref._____

Figure 4. AMA Registry on Adverse Reactions, 1966. (From Council on Drugs, "Reporting Adverse Drug Reactions," Journal of the American Medical Association *196 [2 May 1966]: 144B)*

Most obviously, the possible causes for an adverse reaction ranged across categories of age, race, interaction with other drugs, or even specific batches of a drug. The Council on Drugs did identify several instances of manufacturing accidents and mislabeled drugs. "Spontaneous" reports, however, failed to provide insight into cases that involved multiple drugs or unusual symptoms. More often than not, committee members failed to identify a single causal agent.

The AMA's attempt to centralize and standardize reports on side effects encountered both practical and methodological difficulties. First, members of the committee suspected that physicians only reported a fraction of side effects. Yet neither the committee nor the Council on Drugs had any means by which they could assess how many adverse reactions went unreported, or how many physicians failed to send in forms. As a professional association, the AMA had no mechanism or authority to enforce data collection. Second, AMA committees could not determine how many patients had taken a questionable drug. Efforts to calculate risk profiles were hampered because reports of side effects produced a numerator without a denominator. In other words, the council could not calculate the incidence or frequency of adverse reactions. Council reports reflect frustration with this aspect of its work, and members complained that "physicians reported only a small fraction of all cases and the total number of patients receiving a drug was unknown."[12]

Organizational difficulties also plagued the council's efforts. As an internal memo later noted, the council never assembled a user-friendly database to warn physicians or patients about dangerous drugs. Instead of preempting the spread of adverse reactions, the registry largely collected case reports post-hoc from medical journals and manufacturers. A critical retrospective argued: "In no instance was an adverse reaction reported to the Registry that had not already been observed elsewhere. The reports were entirely unevaluated; there was no follow-up by qualified staff from the AMA. The Registry . . . did not serve as an early warning system."[13]

Council members were unable to force doctors to report side effects. As a result, the registry received case reports from only 2 percent of American physicians.[14] An effort was made to build a voluntary network among doctors in private practice through direct correspondence, publications in widely read journals, and dissemination of forms in *JAMA*. But the council did little to standardize or compare the reports it received. Instead, members discussed each report as an independent case during committee meetings. While the Council on Drugs did assemble a cadre of physicians with practical experience and broad medical expertise, it lacked the organizational structure, financial support, and regulatory authority necessary to operate a successful warning system about drugs on the market.

Enter the FDA

The FDA launched a registry of adverse reactions following enactment of the 1962 Kefauver-Harris Amendments. Unlike the AMA's effort to convince doctors in private practices to submit reports, the FDA initiated its adverse reaction program by collecting data from government-affiliated hospitals. Within a few years, the agency expanded its network to include university clinics and large private hospitals. Initially, the agency gave hospitals broad leeway concerning the format of reports. Starting with a 1966 seminar on Adverse Reactions, however, the FDA promoted a standardized Drug Experience Form.[15] During the meeting, FDA officials explained in detail how to record side effects so that reports were more amenable to statistical analysis.

At the time, hospitals participating in the FDA effort sent in approximately 3,000 reports each month. One-third of these either lacked key data, or were "impossible" to read, code, and analyze. According to FDA officials, better-trained physicians would submit more comprehensive reports: "The physician at the bedside must be able to convey on paper for the Food and Drug physician everything he can about drug use, dose and duration of exposure, time of use, and known toxicity."[16] Unlike the broad sweep of patient information collected by the AMA, the FDA reduced data collection to specifics about medications. In particular, the agency focused on the dose and duration of exposure to a particular drug.

During the 1960s, the FDA and the AMA divided the territory of data collection and analysis. Whereas the federal agency collected reports from Army, Navy, Public Health Service, and Veterans hospitals, the medical profession collected data from smaller hospitals and clinics, as well as doctors operating private practices.[17] FDA officials collaborated with the Council on Drugs and sought to promote greater physician involvement. A 1965 FDA brochure thus admonished doctors to "Report Drug Reactions!" and suggested that an alert and ethically responsible physician would submit reports to the AMA.[18] In the coming years, however, the FDA increased the number of hospitals affiliated with its adverse reactions program, while the AMA saw a steady decline in reports to the Committee on Adverse Reactions.

Converging on the Hospital

The AMA discontinued its nascent registry of adverse reactions in 1970 and launched a Pilot Drug Surveillance Study in an effort to compile information that was more amenable to comparative analysis. Unable to recruit physicians as reliable data collectors, council members mimicked the FDA and turned to hospitals as a more controlled setting. The pilot study's objectives explained this shift as part of an effort to carry out more thorough and systematic research on marketed drugs: "Although the input to the Registry was theoretically much larger than that for the Drug Surveillance Study, in reality the latter will provide much more information since prescribing physicians in each study hospital must report whether or not there was an adverse effect for each standing drug order."[19] Council members anticipated that it would be easier to discipline hospital-based physicians than getting doctors in smaller clinics or private practices to complete and return forms. In addition, the hospital setting guaranteed patient participation, since they could not simply discontinue drug therapy without providing an explanation to their doctors.

When the AMA first developed the Committee on Adverse Reactions, members had hoped to create a national registry that would collect reports and disseminate practical information back to doctors. The Council on Drugs intended for the registry to provide an alternative to the glowing reports found in industry advertising materials. Members wanted to position the AMA as a regulatory body to oversee medicine in the United States. Between its start in 1953 and demise in 1970, however, the registry collected only 8,200 reports, one-third of which related to its original focus on blood dyscrasias. The Council on Drugs succeeded in bringing together respected experts from various medical disciplines to compile and examine this body of data. Nevertheless, AMA officials, council members, and committee participants all found it difficult to convince practicing physicians to submit reports of adverse reactions.

Throughout, council members suspected that a majority of patients failed to inform their physicians of side effects. In response to this perception of a recalcitrant and independent patient, the council turned from "spontaneous" case reports to the more controlled hospital setting. This put the AMA in direct competition with the FDA, which mobilized greater financial resources and expertise with statistical approaches derived from its efforts to standardize clinical trials. While the FDA was later criticized for failing to build contacts with physicians in private practice, it did establish a solid network of data collectors at large teaching hospitals and government clinics during the 1960s. Agency officials used hospital physicians to provide uniform data sets, in part because their patients were considered reliable informants. The hospital thus served as a clinical trial surrogate that integrated testing and monitoring with patient care.

The Federal Chamber of Physicians

In Germany, the medical profession likewise established a central site for collecting information about marketed drugs in the early part of the twentieth century. Physicians were initially motivated by the enormous number of new medicinal compounds produced by dye and chemical companies along with unscrupulous drug compounders. Doctors at the 1911 Congress for Internal Medicine also feared that insurance firms were planning to set fees for services and limit reimbursements for prescription drugs. Physicians voted to create a Drug Commission (Arzneimittelkommission) to provide "objective" information about medicines.[20] Commission leaders sought to position their organization as a gatekeeper between patients and drug producers. They also set criteria for drug quality and safety that preempted a similar move by insurance firms.

The commission soon established a standing committee of clinicians and pharmacologists to examine medications and determine if drugs actually contained the ingredients listed on their packages. Based on laboratory and clinical tests, commission members ranked drugs positive, negative, or dubious, thereby passing judgment on therapeutic efficacy and safety.[21] They then published lists of drugs falling in each category. In this manner, the Drug Commission exercised control over the pharmaceutical industry while simultaneously taking steps to influence drug prescriptions.

Following the 1923 expansion of the Drug Commission from an ancillary organization of the Society for Internal Medicine into a general commission for physicians and insurers, it began producing a comprehensive compendium of medicines recommended for different diseases. Similar to the AMA council, the Drug Commission defined testing standards and recommended specific drugs to treat medical conditions. Starting in 1925, the group published a volume of approved drugs and their precise pharmacological contents, titled *Arzneiverordnungen* (Drug Prescriptions). Only medicines whose "healing power and safety has been sufficiently tested, whose composition is precisely known, and for which claims concerning the origin, composition, and contents are true" were listed in this publication.[22] The Drug Commission thereby asserted a monopoly over drug testing and "objective" information about medications.

Manufacturers still marketed drugs directly to physicians and the public. At the same time, most were willing to pay fees up to 200 Marks for the commission to test their products and list them in its publications. Yet commission members did not have the regulatory authority to remove dangerous drugs from the market. By coupling their testing labs and monitoring of patients with a publication found on every doctor's bookshelf, they nevertheless were able to exert a significant influence on the drug market during the 1920s and early 1930s.

The 1933 Nazi political coordinating act (*Gleichschaltung*) eliminated the rights of churches, schools, universities, the press, and trade unions to set standards and regulate markets. In the medical sector, the law transferred authority over membership criteria, licensing standards, and professional norms from the medical chamber to the national government. Another law prohibited

Jewish physicians from treating patients in hospitals or medical facilities that received government support. The Nazi government next banned publication of the *Arzneiverordnungen*. A central health ministry now declared which medicines could be prescribed by physicians and reimbursed by insurers. In response to these measures, the Drug Commission moved back under the control of the Society for Internal Medicine and discontinued its independent laboratory and clinical drug tests.

Reasserting Professional Authority

Almost immediately following the Allied victory in Europe and the collapse of the Nazi government in Germany, physicians reestablished associations in the western occupation zones. These chambers adopted self-governing (*Selbstverwaltung*) standards for patient care, physician education, and licensing for private practices. Occupying forces in the West supported physicians' efforts to govern the health care market and permitted regional and eventually a national organization to form in West Germany.[23] Doctor Neuffer, head of the Working Group of the West German Chamber of Physicians, proposed in 1950 to broaden the Drug Commission's mandate to address drug safety concerns of the entire medical profession. After his plan was approved in 1952, the Drug Commission of the Federal Chamber of Physicians (Arzneimittelkommission der deutschen Ärzteschaft, or AkdÄ) began carrying out pharmacological, chemical, serological, bacteriological, and clinical experiments on pharmaceutical preparations. The group also issued a new edition of the *Arzneiverordnungen*.

AkdÄ recruited members from university hospitals, private clinics, and general practice. Although not tied to any one spectacular disaster like anemia cases from chloramphenicol use in the United States, concerns about adverse reactions drew increasing attention in Germany during the late 1950s. Beginning with its 1958 annual report, AkdÄ asked practicing physicians to report side effects.[24] The widely read medical journal, *Deutsches Ärzteblatt*, served as the commission's primary means of contacting physicians. Editorials and review essays disseminated information about drug risks. While commission leaders noted chloramphenicol as a particular concern, AkdÄ also warned of medicines containing radioactive elements, overuse of appetite suppressants, and addiction to sedatives found in over-the-counter products, such as lollipops that contained Phenobarbital.

Warnings about sedatives proved prescient once the thalidomide tragedy unfolded in the early 1960s. AkdÄ leaders then expanded their efforts to collect and evaluate reports of adverse reactions from physicians across the country. In order to do so, they published guidelines asking physicians to provide case descriptions of "undesired" reactions to individual drugs or combinations of medicines.[25] As the magnitude of the thalidomide tragedy became apparent, AkdÄ developed a formal system for Spontaneous Reports of Undesired Drug Effects (*Spontanerfassungssystem für unerwünschte Arzneimittelwirkungen*).

Physicians could submit reports on a standardized form (Figure 5) published in the *Deutsches Ärzteblatt* starting in 1963.[26] After compiling and analyzing reports, AkdÄ reported to the medical profession through its Drug Information Service (Arzneimittelinformationsdienst). According to the commission's 1965 Annual Report, new methods of communication among physicians would "make a tragedy like that of thalidomide recognizable more quickly, thereby limiting its scope."[27]

Similar to the AMA Council on Drugs, AkdÄ collected information about patients' age, sex, and diseases, as well as laboratory findings from blood, urine, or other tests. Unlike the AMA, however, AkdÄ asked for fewer precise data points and depended more on physicians' judgments of the seriousness of an adverse reaction. German physicians were asked to list suspected causes of side effects as well as the affected body system. They did not, however, have to list every drug a patient had taken in the last six months, or describe all potentially toxic agents to which patients were exposed. Instead, physicians encountered a series of questions about the course of an adverse reaction (*Verlauf*), how long a patient suffered (*Dauer*), and whether or not the side effect was reversible (*Reversibilität*). In effect, German physicians could give a qualitative assessment of a patient's experience, whereas American doctors had to list (or check off) very specific information about the patient and describe diagnostic methods and treatment measures. German physicians consequently took a more active role in completing forms than their American counterparts.

During the mid-1960s, AkdÄ created a central registry for adverse reactions and established administrative offices and testing labs. It also expanded its network of contacts among practicing physicians and university-based researchers. The commission mobilized this network to forge consensus about which drugs were safe and which were dangerous. Operating as a branch of the larger Chamber of Physicians, AkdÄ could quickly disseminate information to practicing doctors. Like the AMA, however, AkdÄ found it difficult to generalize reports from a small number of cases to general drug therapy.[28] In order to create a more substantial database, AkdÄ turned to hospitals and physicians in large clinics. Commission leaders contacted hospital directors and argued for the importance of a central database despite differences in treatment approaches, drug doses, and routes of drug administration (i.e., intravenous rather than pills) between stationary and ambulatory care.[29] Beyond providing additional data on side effects, hospital-based physicians helped expand the AkdÄ network of "experts beyond its immediate members that are ready to assist in the clarification of urgent and problematic questions."[30]

Bitte um Mitarbeit aller Ärzte:

Unverträglichkeit oder Nebenwirkungen von Arzneimitteln melden!

Die rasch fortschreitende Entwicklung hat zu einer großen Erweiterung der arzneitherapeutischen Möglichkeiten geführt. Die Erfahrung hat aber gezeigt, daß auch sorgfältigste experimentelle und klinische Prüfung neuer Arzneimittel noch nicht einen vollständigen Überblick über alle nur möglichen Nebenwirkungen gewährleisten kann. Manche Unverträglichkeiten und Nebenwirkungen werden erst bei breiter Anwendung in der ärztlichen Praxis bemerkt oder können in ihrer Bedeutung und Häufigkeit dann erst richtig beurteilt werden.

Um Gefahren durch Arzneimittel möglichst frühzeitig erkennen und die Ärzteschaft unterrichten zu können, werden alle Ärzte zur Mitarbeit aufgerufen!

Die Bundesärztekammer und ihre Arzneimittelkommission bitten alle Ärzte dringend, ihre Beobachtungen über Unverträglichkeiten oder Nebenwirkungen eines Arzneimittels — besonders eines neuen — oder auch den bloßen V e r d a c h t auf Nebenwirkungen der Arzneimittelkommission der Deutschen Ärzteschaft mitzuteilen. Benutzen Sie bitte untenstehenden Vordruck.

Nur die Sammlung aller Beobachtungen an einer zentralen Stelle ermöglicht die frühzeitige Erkennung von Gefahren.

·· Bitte hier abtrennen ··

An die Arzneimittelkommission der Deutschen Ärzteschaft
(Ausschuß der Bundesärztekammer)
34 Göttingen, Bunsenstraße 11

Betr.: Unverträglichkeit oder Nebenwirkungen von Arzneimitteln
(Bitte auch Fälle von Verdacht mitteilen!)

Bitte füllen Sie dieses Formular aus, soweit es den Umständen nach möglich ist.

Patient (chiffriert):   männlich / weiblich   Geburtsdatum: _____ Wohnort: _____

Diagnose: _____

_____

Therapeutische Maßnahmen: _____
(alle verordneten Medikamente möglichst mit Dosierung)

_____

Welchem Mittel werden die Nebenwirkungen zugeschrieben? (Dosierung?): _____

Art der Erscheinungen: (Haut, Herz-Kreislauf, Magen-Darm, Atmungsorgane, Zentralnervensystem, Sinnesorgane, Muskulatur, Sonstiges?)

_____

Verlauf? _____

Dauer? _____

Reversibilität? _____

Krankenhauseinweisung ja / nein   Welches Krankenhaus?: _____

Anamnestische Angaben: _____

Allergiker? _____

Besondere Krankheiten oder besondere Therapie in der Anamnese? _____

_____

Laborbefunde (falls vorhanden) über Blut? Urin? Stuhl? _____

_____

Sonstige Bemerkungen: _____

_____

Figure 5. AkdÄ reporting form, 1964. (From Deutsches Ärzteblatt, 1964)

Responding to Drug Disasters

The networked approach followed by AkdÄ confined concerns about side effects to a narrow community of experts, even in the wake of well-publicized drug disasters. Rather than becoming grounds for citizen mobilization for greater federal protection, cases of serious adverse reactions instead served to shore up the authority of the medical profession. Specifically, the Drug Commission used instances of high-profile side effects to demonstrate its ability to restrict the use of dangerous drugs without making them completely unavailable to patients who could benefit from them.

In the chloramphenicol case, German physicians initially responded to events in the United States. The FDA severely restricted the use of this antibiotic in 1968, following years of debates regarding its link to aplastic anemia and fatal blood dyscrasias. AkdÄ then carried out a survey of its members to study the frequency of chloramphenicol-related side effects in Germany. After tabulating responses, the commission found that rates of aplastic anemia and fatal blood dyscrasias were significantly lower than in the United States. Reacting less stringently than the FDA, AkdÄ suggested that physicians reduce the dosage and shorten the length of prescriptions.

AkdÄ thus acted to influence physicians in a subtler manner than a formal ban. As commissioners argued, "With this advice, necessary boundaries are established within which chloramphenicol can be used, without having to abandon this generally valuable—and for the treatment of certain diseases, indispensable—antibiotic."[31] At the same time that AkdÄ set "boundaries" for chloramphenicol use, it also demarcated its authority as distinct from a state-based regulatory body. Operating by consensus among a network of medical professionals, it could circumscribe medical practices and shield patients from dangerous drugs.

An association between the appetite suppressant Menocil and heart damage provided AkdÄ with a second case where it could achieve regulation by means of professional consensus. The Swiss firm Cilag contacted AkdÄ about cases of pulmonary hypertension (abnormally elevated blood pressure) related to Menocil in August 1968. The German Drug Commission initially replied that it had no reports on file connecting their drug to hypertension. Nevertheless, based on correspondence with the Swiss medical association and further communication with the company, AkdÄ and Cilag sent out a joint letter warning over 100,000 German physicians of the potential for Menocil to cause heart damage. A year later, AkdÄ reported that it still lacked sufficient evidence to prove a causal relationship between Menocil and hypertension, even though it had collected seventy reports of side effects. AkdÄ nevertheless sent another letter warning physicians not to prescribe the drug, except to severely obese patients. Officials also stressed that physicians should monitor patients taking the drug to ensure that they followed the treatment regimen closely.[32]

In the meantime, newspaper, radio, and television reports drew public attention to the case. Many reports drew analogies between Menocil and the thalidomide disaster, thereby implicating the medical profession and AkdÄ in a close and "dangerous" alliance with drug companies.[33] Responding to criticisms that the Drug Commission failed to act quickly enough in these cases, AkdÄ drew a division between its role as a professional organization and the role of government regulatory agencies found in other countries.

The commission explained that it operated as a voluntary advisory body in the absence of a national regulatory agency in Germany: "The Drug Commission is not an agency similar to the FDA or the state regulatory commissions of other countries; it was created for physicians through the self-initiative of the medical profession and has taken on a series of tasks that are often the responsibility of government departments in other countries."[34] Asserting that they had filled the gap created by an absence of federal regulations, AkdÄ leaders nevertheless claimed that the commission served as an attentive observer, not regulator, of the pharmaceutical market.

Controversy and public attention to the thalidomide, chloramphenicol, and Menocil cases helped motivate physicians to collect reports about adverse reactions. In turn, AkdÄ acted as a central node in the network by compiling data and reporting to physicians. Participation in the flow of information was controlled tightly. Based on a construction of "the patient" as fearful of even life-saving medicines in the wake of drug tragedies, the Drug Commission explicitly avoided "causing public alarm by involving open forms of communication (press, television, radio)."[35] Instead, AkdÄ mailed information directly to physicians with a large red hand printed on the envelope, along with the text "important information."[36] The organization defended its refusal to warn the public directly by claiming, "No sick person is aided when distrust is raised concerning potentially life-saving medicines prescribed by physicians in a responsible manner."[37] Members of the Drug Commission thus sought to maintain a body of professional knowledge by controlling information and preventing patients from learning about drug risks from sources other than their physicians.

Widely reported cases of adverse drug reactions fueled suspicions in Germany that the medical profession and drug companies masked other cases of side effects. Starting in the late 1960s, the German parliament pressured the Federal Health Office (Bundesgesundheitsamt, or BGA) to exercise greater control over the drug market. In response, BGA officials formed a scientific working group on the "Safety of Drugs" in 1969. Not surprisingly, AkdÄ criticized this group as redundant, bureaucratically inefficient, and a potentially harmful duplication of its activities. At the same time that the FDA was developing an in-house division responsible for collecting, tallying, and responding to side effects, the BGA also turned its attention to the issue. In contrast to developments in the United States, however, the German agency did not advance beyond pulling together an advisory group. Despite criticisms of close ties between the medical profession and the pharmaceutical industry, AkdÄ retained its monopoly role over a network of physicians that collected and responded to adverse reactions.

Data Collection in Different Therapeutic Cultures

Unlike the AMA's failed efforts to catalog side effects, AkdÄ established a stable network for exchanging information about marketed drugs. The Federal Chamber of Physicians claimed not to occupy a regulatory role; nevertheless it sought to prevent the government from assuming greater authority over the drug market. In effect, the widely accepted construction of the patient as someone needing guidance and protection by medical professionals helped AkdÄ avoid crossing over from professional association to regulatory authority. Patient autonomy and reluctance to participate in postmarket data collection were not as significant as in the United States. AkdÄ contributed to the apparently widely held view that patients needed professional supervision by coordinating a network of physicians in private practices, hospitals, and universities that shared information with each other and pharmaceutical manufacturers. This system ultimately diffused blame for side effects and other medical disasters across the network, thereby shielding experts from public scrutiny, criticism, and accountability.

In contrast to the German situation, the AMA and FDA offered competing political constructions of the patient during the 1950s and 1960s. Whereas the AMA Council on Drugs wanted to protect autonomous individuals from potentially dangerous medicines, FDA officials calculated risk factors for broader patient populations and then informed physicians and consumers about drug safety. Both organizations agreed that the majority of patients were unreliable data sources about marketed drugs. They therefore turned to hospitals as controlled sites for data collection. Once the FDA took over as the peak regulatory authority for adverse reactions, it provided a locus for public scrutiny and demands for government accountability. Ironically, regulatory centralization ultimately contributed to greater transparency and better information flow to the public in the United States than was found in the more decentralized and networked German system.

State Authority and Medical Associations, 1970–2000

By the early 1970s, therapeutic cultures of the United States and Germany markedly diverged, notably in these countries' institutional responses to side effects. Concerns about misleading industry advertising and drug tragedies had led the U.S. Congress to protect "unwitting consumers" by imposing safety and efficacy standards. Likewise, FDA fears about the political ramifications of approved drugs that caused adverse reactions led the agency to focus on controlled clinical trials as the gold standard for premarket testing. Once drugs were on the market, unease about the reliability of "autonomous individuals" led the FDA to use hospitals as a controlled environment for data collection. In contrast, the German Bundestag largely left the protection of patients "frightened" by drug tragedies in the hands of the medical profession. The BGA was assigned little authority to enforce specific methods for clinical trials or to collect information about drugs on the market. Instead, AkdÄ oversaw a network of medical professionals and company representatives that balanced cases of drug disasters against the needs of patients with a variety of diseases.

Because of these differences, the United States adopted an all-or-nothing approach to regulatory approvals and postmarket review, whereas Germany took a more nuanced position that restricted the use of dangerous drugs without completely banning them. During the next three decades, these two systems for drug regulation had to respond to important changes in each country's therapeutic culture. Patient activists and disease-based organizations in the United States took a more aggressive role in defining the patient's needs and challenged the FDA's precautionary approach. Consequently, the agency approved drugs more quickly. FDA officials then turned greater attention to postmarket studies and even began accepting reports of side effects directly from patients. In contrast, German physicians maintained their key position in the network of organizations overseeing the drug market. While the BGA and its successor institute, BfArM, expanded their authority in response to pressures from the European Union, fewer major changes were evident in German constructions of the patient's position in the therapeutic network during the 1980s and 1990s.

State-Based Pharmacovigilance in the United States

Like the AMA's Council on Drugs, the FDA initially found it difficult to convince physicians and hospital administrators to submit reports of adverse reactions. FDA officials resolved issues of data analysis that plagued the AMA by developing formal methods to codify and compare reports of adverse reactions. Agency officials soon recognized that too much data in a given case complicated drawing causal connections between individual drugs and specific reactions. Simplified reporting forms that reduced the number of possible confounding factors, however, might not prompt physicians to record crucial evidence.

Officials at the FDA Bureau of Medicines debated this dilemma: "It has been found that if the case-reporting format is sufficiently comprehensive to include all of the items which are desired, it becomes so involved that cooperation and interest in the reporting of individual cases will rapidly diminish."[38] As a compromise, they devised a Drug Experience Report that combined key elements of the AMA reporting form with concerns that had arisen in the early 1960s.

The new reporting form (Figure 6) did not ask hospital-based physicians to provide significantly different data than requested by the AMA. Like the Council on Drugs, the FDA sought to correlate drug-induced side effects with data on patient age, weight, and racial group. Unlike the AMA, the FDA included a new category for information about pregnant women, reflecting post-thalidomide sensibilities about birth defects. The agency did not require physicians to provide their names, although it did request the "source" of each report. The AMA had collected information about physicians as part of an effort to shape their prescribing patterns and therapeutic practices. The FDA was more interested in where a report originated than in the individual physician who identified an adverse reaction. Along these same lines, the FDA asked for "existing or prior disorders and past drug reaction or allergic history," rather than collect information about other drugs taken during the past six months. Changes to the reporting form thus reflect a larger shift: from the AMA acting as a gatekeeper between physicians and drug companies to the FDA mediating between patients and the pharmaceutical industry.

Above and beyond changes to reporting forms, administrative controls more readily available to the FDA than the AMA helped ensure that physicians completed the paperwork. Hospitals participating in the adverse reaction reporting system were required to designate a program coordinator. The coordinator instructed physicians about collection practices and reviewed reports before sending them to the government. Hospitals that observed at least two hundred patients were paid a monthly stipend of $200 in 1969, regardless of the number of reports they collected.[39] Because of these disciplining features and modest financial incentives, the FDA soon received some 1,000 case reports each month from participating hospitals. These were supplemented by additional reports from drug companies.

Translating and Standardizing Reports

In order to evaluate and draw conclusions from this mass of data, the agency developed a standardized medical terminology and codified reports

Figure 6.
FDA Drug
Experience Report,
1967. (FDA Archives/
Records Office)

DEPARTMENT OF
HEALTH, EDUCATION, AND WELFARE
FOOD AND DRUG ADMINISTRATION
WASHINGTON, D.C. 20204

DRUG EXPERIENCE REPORT

BUDGET BUREAU NO. 57–R0004
Approval Expires December 31, 1970

DATE SENT TO FDA
(Mo, day, yr)
1. ☐ INITIAL REPORT
☐ FOLLOW UP REPORT

2. PATIENT INITIALS AND IDENTIFICATION NUMBER

3. ACCESSION NO. (For FDA use only)

SECTION I. BASIC REACTION DATA

4. SEX ☐ M ☐ F

5. HEIGHT ___ Ins.

WEIGHT ___ lbs.

6. DATE OF BIRTH ___ mo ___ day ___ yr

7. ORIGIN ☐ CAUC ☐ NEGRO ☐ ORIENTAL ☐ AMERICAN INDIAN ☐ OTHER

8. DATE OF REACTION ONSET ___ mo ___ day ___ yr

9. SOURCE OF REPORT (Mfg. Hospital, etc) (Name of reporting Physician is optional.)

10. ADDRESS OF SOURCE (Give Street, City, State, and Zip Code.)

11. DESCRIBE SUSPECTED ADVERSE REACTION(s) AND ANY POSSIBLE ASSOCIATION WITH THE DRUG(s) INVOLVED

12. OUTCOME OF REACTION TO DATE
☐ ALIVE WITH SEQUELAE
☐ RECOVERED
☐ STILL UNDER TREATMENT
☐ DIED (Give date and cause)

13. LIST ALL THERAPY IN ORDER OF SUSPICION (Manufacturer; List NDA or IND No.)

NAME OF DRUGS TRADE (Generic)	MANUFACTURERS CONTROL NO.	DOSAGE FORM (tab, cap, etc.)	TOTAL DAILY DOSE	ROUTE (po, im, iv, etc.)	DURATION # OF THERAPY	DATES OF ADMINISTRATION	14. DISORDER OR REASON FOR USE OF DRUG

SECTION II. IMPORTANT MODIFYING DATA

15. SUBSTANTIATING LABORATORY STUDIES (Clinical Laboratory, Autopsy, X-Ray, etc.)

CLINICAL LAB: ☐ DONE ☐ ATTACHED ☐ NOT DONE

BIOPSY/AUTOPSY: ☐ DONE ☐ ATTACHED ☐ NOT DONE

16. LIST POTENTIALLY NOXIOUS OR ENVIRONMENTAL FACTORS (Include household products, industrial and agricultural chemicals)

17. EXISTING OR PRIOR DISORDERS AND PAST DRUG REACTION OR ALLERGIC HISTORY

PREVIOUS EXPOSURE TO SUSPECTED DRUG OR RELATED COMPOUND ☐ YES ☐ NO

18. (a) IF FEMALE
GRAVIDITY ___ PARITY ___

(b) IF PREGNANT
WEEKS OF GESTATION ___

19. MAY THE SOURCE OF THIS REPORT BE RELEASED TO THE ARMED FORCES INSTITUTE OF PATHOLOGY? ☐ YES ☐ NO

FOR FDA USE ONLY

20. REACTION FACTORS (Check all applicable boxes)
☐ DECOMPOSITION OF DRUG ☐ INTERACTION OF TWO OR MORE DRUGS ☐ DRUG NOT USED ACCORDING TO LABELING ☐ DRUG OUTDATED
☐ DRUG MISUSED BY PATIENT ☐ OVERDOSAGE ☐ DRUG MISLABELED ☐ CONTAMINATION OF DRUG ☐ OTHER DRUG MISUSE (specify)

FOR MFG USE ONLY

FORM FD–1639 (Rev 8/67)

SEE INSTRUCTIONS ON REVERSE

Use additional sheet if necessary.

accordingly. The FDA grouped adverse reactions into one of sixteen primary categories, based on individual organs or biological systems. Medical officers also could select among twenty-two secondary categories to describe impacts on patients, such as addiction or withdrawal symptoms. In effect, FDA employees carried out what science studies scholars have termed a "translation" activity.[40] They translated information from diverse physicians' reports of adverse reactions to fit with a fixed set of categories. By this process, the FDA became the central site for responding to side effects. As Bruno Latour explains, translation "refers to all the displacements through other actors whose mediation is indispensable for any action to occur."[41] When culling information for databases from field reports, the FDA made decisions analogous to those of AMA or AkdÄ. Unlike physicians at these medical associations, however, FDA employees followed codified and formalized rules for data entry. Decisions about specific drugs were consequently based less upon expert judgment than on formal routines for converting and comparing reports from the field.

For the FDA, this process of translation and data conversion produced numerical data about the severity of any given reaction. Once entered into computerized databases, this data laid the foundation for comparative and statistical evaluations. In the American context, only the translation from physician's report to a statistical data set allowed patterns to emerge. Officials designed their computer system so that searches could examine medicines and adverse reactions over time or by body system.

Describing some key aspects of this process, one official bragged that the agency could "generate reports of all thrombo-embolic events associated with oral contraceptives; sort by trade name of drug; sort by body system categories and specific thrombo-embolic sites; sort by 5-year age groups; sort by year of occurrence."[42] By translating physicians' reports—themselves a translation of patients' experiences into medical terminology—into a set of standard categories, the FDA resolved some of the difficulties in comparing reports encountered by the AMA. These very translations made it possible for the FDA to use reports of side effects to intervene and withdraw dangerous drugs from the market.

Over the course of the next fifteen years, FDA officials expanded the terminology associated with adverse reactions into a complex "dictionary" that could handle wide variability in drug names and different methods for data entry that persisted despite attempts to create bureaucratic uniformity.[43] Intriguingly, the agency's regulatory authority was build upon a regime of numbers. By implementing a quantitative approach for data collection and comparison, the FDA could visibly demonstrate its ability to meet public and congressional demands for drug safety.

Turning Patients into Data Collectors

Just as in clinical trials, patients since the mid-1980s have come to the forefront of discussions about how to best structure the system for reporting and responding to adverse reactions. The FDA expanded its monitoring of adverse reactions as an integral part of efforts to speed drug approvals. Officials blurred the boundary between pre- and postmarket drug evaluation by expanding data collection to include physicians in private practices and even began collecting reports directly from patients through the Internet.

Regulations issued in 1985 created a "Central Document Room" to handle reports of adverse reactions.[44] While the agency had long served as a central site for data collection and analysis for the United States, the new document room visibly centralized this function within the FDA. The 1985 regulations also required manufacturers to share reports with the government within fifteen days. At the same time, FDA officials turned to physicians in private practice, small clinics, and other treatment facilities as sources for more data. Articles in prominent medical journals helped recruit these physicians.[45] According to the FDA, successful policy responses to adverse reactions now hinged on the participation of individual doctors: "FDA monitoring of adverse reactions is primarily based on 'spontaneous' reports from practicing physicians—i.e., reports that originate from observations made in the usual practice of medicine (not derived from a formal study)."[46]

Picking up on criticisms articulated by AIDS activists and other disease-based organizations, the FDA agreed that premarket tests were limited by the participation of patients from narrow demographic bands. Vulnerable individuals, including "women, children, elderly persons, and patients with complicated diseases," tended only to get drugs after their market approval. In order to include marginalized individuals and broader demographic groups in the postmarket data collection regime, the agency began collecting reports from a wider array of practicing physicians.

With the launch of MEDWatch in 1993, the agency embarked on a significant effort to increase awareness of side effects and recruit both physicians and patients to serve as data collectors. In effect, the FDA participated in a shift in the construction of patients—from passive recipients of medical care who need government protection to informed consumers who choose their drugs—by loosening restrictions on premarket testing. At the same time, officials feared that without better monitoring of adverse reactions, this shift in the therapeutic culture could result in another serious drug tragedy.

Initially the MEDWatch program was intended to simplify reporting and enroll more physicians and other health professionals in the process of reporting side effects. According to FDA Commissioner David Kessler, "It is not in the culture of U.S. medicine to notify the FDA about adverse events or product problems."[47] Nevertheless, since the reporting of side effects is not a legal obligation for physicians, it remains very much a "cultural" issue for the agency. Government officials tried to change American medical culture by introducing and publicizing new reporting forms.

The MEDWatch reporting form (Figure 7) builds upon and modifies the earlier FDA Drug Experience Report in several ways. The form has a larger number of boxes that "health professionals" can simply check off, instead of having to write out extensive details. More specifically, patient information has been reduced to a confidential "identifier," generally the patient's initials, and their age, sex, and weight. Race and ethnicity are no longer present as distinct "census" boxes to be checked. Even though both are referred to in debates over drug safety and efficacy, only race appears on the MEDWatch form under "other relevant history," a category that includes allergies, pregnancy, smoking, and alcohol use. Reflecting changes in medical technologies, the form has been expanded to include medical devices, not just prescription drugs. The language of "health professionals" likewise tracks another key change in American medicine. The FDA recognizes that medical care now is distributed among a variety of practitioners and professions. Outcomes of an adverse reaction have been narrowed to six categories, ranging from "death" to an "intervention to prevent permanent damage." Finally, the form includes a legal disclaimer, stating that "submission of a report does not constitute an admission that medical personnel or the product caused or contributed to the event."

Recent changes to the doctor-patient relationship and the therapeutic culture within which it is embedded have compounded the agency's historical difficulties with reports about side effects. Patients billed for every office visit are more likely to simply stop taking a drug than to report problems to physicians. More subtly, the culture of American individualism continues to lionize patients who seek out their own medicines, often through self-diagnosis aided by direct-to-consumer drug advertisements, popular books that narrate successful self-treatment, and extensive Internet discussion groups. According to a survey, one-third of American households look for medical information on the Internet each week.[48] As part of the FDA's website, MEDWatch provides electronic access to reporting forms and offers extensive information about marketed drugs to health professionals, patients, or anyone else.

In a significant change from previous strategies, MEDWatch combines data collection with information and warnings about drugs on the market. Furthermore, it is not targeted exclusively to physicians. Instead, the FDA now accepts reports directly from patients and provides public access to aggregate data on side effects. The agency recommends that patients with serious drug reactions take the MEDWatch form to their doctor. Nevertheless, since "not all patients

MEDWATCH

The FDA Safety Information and Adverse Event Reporting Program

For **VOLUNTARY** reporting of
adverse events and product problems

Form Approved: OMB No. 0910-0230 Expires: 09/30/05
See OMB statement on reverse

FDA Use Only

Triage unit
sequence #

A. Patient information

1. Patient identifier	2. Age at time of event:	3. Sex	4. Weight
Unspecified In confidence	or _____ Date of birth:	☐ female ☐ male	____ lbs or ____ kgs

B. Adverse event or product problem

1. ☐ Adverse event   and/or   ☐ Product problem (e.g., defects/malfunctions)

2. Outcomes attributed to adverse event (check all that apply)
   - ☐ death _____ (mo/day/yr)
   - ☐ life-threatening
   - ☐ hospitalization - initial or prolonged
   - ☐ disability
   - ☐ congenital anomaly
   - ☐ required intervention to prevent permanent impairment/damage
   - ☐ other: _____

3. Date of event (mo/day/yr)	4. Date of this report (mo/day/yr)

5. Describe event or problem

6. Relevant tests/laboratory data, including dates

7. Other relevant history, including preexisting medical conditions (e.g., allergies, race, pregnancy, smoking and alcohol use, hepatic/renal dysfunction, etc.)

C. Suspect medication(s)

1. Name (give labeled strength & mfr/labeler, if known)
   #1
   #2

2. Dose, frequency & route used	3. Therapy dates (if unknown, give duration) from/to (or best estimate)
#1	#1
#2	#2

4. Diagnosis for use (indication)	5. Event abated after use stopped or dose reduced
#1	#1 ☐ yes ☐ no ☐ doesn't apply
#2	#2 ☐ yes ☐ no ☐ doesn't apply

6. Lot # (if known)	7. Exp. date (if known)	8. Event reappeared after reintroduction
#1	#1	#1 ☐ yes ☐ no ☐ doesn't apply
#2	#2	#2 ☐ yes ☐ no ☐ doesn't apply

9. NDC # (for product problems only)

10. Concomitant medical products and therapy dates (exclude treatment of event)

D. Suspect medical device

1. Brand name

2. Type of device

3. Manufacturer name & address	4. Operator of device
	☐ health professional ☐ lay user/patient ☐ other: _____

6.	5. Expiration date (mo/day/yr)
model # _____	
catalog # _____	7. If implanted, give date (mo/day/yr)
serial # _____	
lot # _____	8. If explanted, give date (mo/day/yr)
other #	

9. Device available for evaluation?   (Do not send to FDA)
   ☐ yes   ☐ no   ☐ returned to manufacturer on _____ (mo/day/yr)

10. Concomitant medical products and therapy dates (exclude treatment of event)

E. Reporter (see confidentiality section on back)

1. Name & address	phone #

2. Health professional?	3. Occupation	4. Also reported to
☐ yes ☐ no		☐ manufacturer
5. If you do NOT want your identity disclosed to the manufacturer, place an " X " in this box. ☐		☐ user facility ☐ distributor

---

FDA

Mail to: **MEDWATCH**
5600 Fishers Lane
Rockville, MD 20852-9787

or FAX to:
1-800-FDA-0178

FDA Form 3500 (11/02)   Submission of a report does not constitute an admission that medical personnel or the product caused or contributed to the event.

Figure 7. FDA MEDWatch online voluntary reporting form, contemporary.
(⟨http//www.accessdata.fda.gov/scripts/medwatch/pdf/medwatch.pdf⟩)

feel comfortable discussing side effects with their physicians, or have easy access to doctors," the agency devised a web-based form that the lay public can submit directly.[49] Avoiding direct competition with physicians, the agency does not suggest alternative treatments or offer palliative measures for patients' complaints. Nevertheless, in an era when patients rarely establish long-term relationships with physicians, the FDA offers itself as a trustworthy confidant for intimate medical details. At the same time, it now accepts patients as reliable and trustworthy sources of information about drugs in their bodies.

Contemporary Controversies

The agency continues to face difficulties recruiting physicians and patients to complete forms. Recent drug withdrawals due to side effects have drawn high-level policy attention to data collection methods and sparked a debate about the speed with which the FDA approves new drugs. A study of two hospitals in New York and a meta-analysis of electronic databases both concluded that between 100,000 and 200,000 patients die annually from adverse medical events. Most of these fatalities are associated with pharmaceutical drugs.[50] By these estimates, pharmaceutical drugs are the fourth leading cause of death in the United States.

Specific cases have also attracted a great deal of attention in the past fifteen years. The antiarrhythmic heart medications Tambocor and Enkaid were linked to between 24,000 and 70,000 deaths each year during the late 1980s.[51] More recently, Rezulin, a treatment for type-2 (adult onset) diabetes, was withdrawn after it was linked to at least sixty-three deaths and other cases of life-threatening disabilities.[52] The case drew congressional attention following allegations that the manufacturer, Warner-Lambert, misrepresented clinical data and failed to inform physicians about side effects after Rezulin's 1997 approval. Other drug withdrawals, including the weight-loss treatment Redux, the heartburn drug Propulsid, and the cholesterol inhibitor Baycol, have prompted editorials in medical journals and scathing reviews of the FDA's pre- and postmarket review mechanisms.[53]

These cases also provoked an investigation into FDA policies by the Institute of Medicine (IOM), a division of the National Academy of Sciences. Criticizing the absence of national reporting requirements, the IOM report suggested that hospitals receiving federal Medicare and Medicaid funds should be required to report to the FDA.[54] IOM members also proposed a National Center for Patient Safety that would review drugs on the market and distribute information to physicians and the public.

Concerns about adverse reactions thus have raised questions about the FDA's approval process just as the agency sought to relax its historically strict separation of clinical testing from general marketing. Responding to contradictory political pressures, the agency has built up "sentinel sites" to carry out postmarketing studies in specific areas such as cardiovascular disease or arthritis.[55] By this mechanism, the FDA is further extending clinical trial approaches to the open market. If premarket tests fail to involve a "vulnerable, understudied population, such as children, women, or the elderly," additional observation of patients will fill gaps once a drug is marketed.[56]

In the flurry of recent activity surrounding adverse drug reactions in the United States, the patient has become a far more differentiated and contested category than ever before. Media reports, including investigations by journalists at the *New York Times* and *Los Angeles Times*, present a public in need of government protection from dangerous drugs and profit-oriented drug companies. These reports frequently portray patients as innocent "guinea pigs," a comparison similar to that made in the Kefauver era described in Chapter 2. The FDA, on the other hand, has moved beyond a discourse of protection to view patients as consumers who need information in order to make rational choices. It thus expends less effort on patrolling the boundary between testing and market than on monitoring and reviewing data about medicines even after they are marketed. In turn, the agency is working to disseminate information to the public on the Internet and through print media.

Categories of "underrepresented minorities" and "vulnerable populations" that patient activists brought to the fore in debates over clinical trials thus shaped regulatory practices for the postmarketing arena as well. Nevertheless, as recent criticisms of the agency document, drugs that produce life-threatening side effects also generate serious political risks to the agency, despite an advanced degree of patient involvement in the production of data on medical risks and transparency of the FDA decision-making process.

Networked Pharmacovigilance in Germany

The network of organizations responsible for monitoring the German drug market faced fewer external critics between 1970 and the present than the more centralized FDA. Cooperation between the Federal Health Ministry and the Drug Commission during the early 1970s helped solidify AkdÄ's role in collecting and standardizing reports of adverse reactions. Following implementation of the 1976 Drug Law in 1978, the government shifted from merely providing an additional forum for discussing side effects to a more active role monitoring the drug market. Specifically, the BGA implemented the "step-plan" (*Stufenplan*), a formal procedure for information exchange and risk management. AkdÄ was included in the *Stufenplan* from the start, has maintained and regularly updated its registry of adverse reactions, and continues to inform physicians about drug risks. The balance of power among industry, government, and the medical profession was challenged in the early 1990s when a drug manufacturer sued AkdÄ for publicizing adverse reactions. The German network nevertheless proved resilient to major changes, even when faced with publicity about unsafe drugs on the market or legal disputes between pharmaceutical manufacturers and the Drug Commission.

Cooperation between AkdÄ and the BGA was cemented in 1970 when Georg Henneberg, a member of the commission since 1952, became president of the BGA. Under his leadership, the two organizations exchanged data on side effects, held joint meetings on problem drugs, and nurtured contacts between physicians and the medical officers responsible for registering new drugs at the BGA. Collaboration with the government did not, however, change the methods used by AkdÄ to evaluate reports of side effects. Members of the Drug Commission recognized the importance of standardizing reports in order to gain comparative perspectives. Unlike the FDA, however, they staunchly defended qualitative assessments as equal or even superior to statistical compilations.

For example, an influential AkdÄ member argued in 1971 that without an impossibly strict data-gathering regime, no method could assess reports of side effects relative to the frequency with which specific drugs were prescribed. Furthermore, rare adverse reactions—precisely because of their infrequency—were not amenable to quantitative analysis. He explained, "For that reason the Drug Commission bypasses criteria found in statistical methods and uses primarily qualitative approaches when evaluating reported observations."[57] Despite attention by federal authorities to side effects, AkdÄ continued to determine methods for reporting, standardizing, and reviewing reports of adverse reactions. Qualitative analysis by experts using a case-by-case method emerged as the premier approach for evaluating medicines on the German market.

As part of the 1976 Drug Law, the BGA took on responsibility for creating a national registry of adverse drug reactions. Officials incorporated reports from AkdÄ, pharmaceutical companies, pharmacists, and other sources. Though intended to supersede the medical profession, the government registry depended heavily on AkdÄ members to provide the expertise necessary to integrate disparate data sets and evaluate reports. The newly created Institute for Drugs (Arzneimittelinstitut) at the BGA did not assert a strong regulatory stance over postmarketing drug evaluation. Instead, institute leaders exchanged reports with AkdÄ and followed its consensus-based approach to governing the drug market. Rather than force withdrawals, for example, they collaborated with physicians and manufacturers to establish more uniform prescribing methods and recommend safer dosages of harmful drugs.

Karl Überla, president of the BGA in the early 1980s, worried about the absence of government-driven standardization and the failure to quantify adverse reaction reports in Germany. During a 1983 conference on the role of the government in ensuring drug safety, he recommended major changes to data collection and review.[58] First and foremost, Überla wanted to implement a standardized terminology to categorize side effects. In turn, formal algorithms would determine their significance. He also advised both the Institute for Drugs and AkdÄ to carry out systematic randomized tests of marketed drugs, calculate the frequency of side effects under different conditions, and ensure that observations were independent, reproducible, and unbiased. Überla's desire to quantify drug risks, however, ran up against the long-standing tradition of professional assessment on a case-by-case approach. As a result, the BGA implemented few of his proposals.

Sharing Secrets

The BGA instead developed formal procedures for sharing information among industry, the medical profession, and the government. By implementing the *Stufenplan* for risk mitigation during the 1980s, the BGA gradually structured reporting and response mechanisms into a closed web of expertise similar to methods followed in clinical trials and the review of new drug applications. Information flow within the network was codified in 1986 Amendments to the German Drug Law. Under the revised law, pharmaceutical firms had to dedicate staff to the *Stufenplan*, and professional associations—including AkdÄ and its counterpart for the pharmacy profession—were listed as sources for expert analysis.[59] In practice, AkdÄ has played a far more active role than simply giving advice when consulted. Instead, commission leaders expanded and computerized their database and continue to encourage physicians to report side effects directly to the organization on a revised form.

Unlike earlier reporting forms used in Germany, the new AkdÄ form (Figure 8) asks physicians to disaggregate information about the patient and the patient's disease, treatments, and adverse reaction. Physicians first are requested to provide the patient's initials, date of birth, sex, height, weight, occupation, ethnicity, and whether or not they were pregnant. Next, they are asked to describe the side effects, when they occurred, and how long they lasted. Third, doctors can list up to four drugs, their dosage, application form, and dates of administration as well as why they were prescribed. Suspected associations between these treatments and the adverse reaction are indicated by checking a box, "Vermuteter Zusammenhang mit Arzneimittel-Nr."

Potentially confounding variables come next, and physicians can mark off items ranging from nicotine to drug abuse. Much as in the United States, they are asked to describe the medical outcome of the side effect. Unlike the FDA

Bericht über unerwünschte Arzneimittelwirkungen (auch Verdachtsfälle)
an die Arzneimittelkommission der deutschen Ärzteschaft (AkdÄ) gemäß der Berufsordnung für Ärzte
Postfach 41 01 25 • 50861 Köln • Telefax: (0221) 4004 -539 • Telefon: (0221) 4004 -512

Pat.Init.	Geburtsdatum	Geschlecht m □ w □	Größe (cm)	Gewicht (kg)	ethn. Zugeh.	Schwangersch.- Monat: __ __
__ __	__ __ __ __ __		__ __ __	__ __ __		

Beobachtete unerwünschte Wirkungen   aufgetreten am: __ __, __ __, __ __   Dauer: __ __ Stunden __ __ Tage

lebensbedrohlich? ja □ nein □

Arzneimittel/Darreichungsform ggf. Chargenbezeichnung	Tagesdosis	Applikation	gegeben von/bis	wegen
①				
②				
③				

Vermuteter Zusammenhang   dieses früher verabreicht   vertragen   ggf. Reexposition
mit Arzneimittel Nr. ① ② ③   ja □ nein □   ja □ nein □   nein □ neg. □ pos. □

Grunderkrankung (ggf. ICD-Codierung):   **Begleiterkrankungen:** (ggf. ICD-Codierung)

Anamn. Besonderheiten, z. B.: Alkohol □ Allergien* □ Arzneimittelabusus* □ Diät □ Implantate □ Kontrazeptiva □ Rauchen □
Sonstige:

* weitere Erläuterungen:

Veränderung von Laborparametern in Zusammenhang mit der unerwünschten Arzneimittelwirkung:

Verlauf und Therapie der unerwünschten Arzneimittelwirkung:

Ausgang der unerwünschten Arzneimittelwirkung:
wiederhergestellt □ wiederhergestellt mit Defekt □ noch nicht wiederhergestellt □ unbekannt □ Exitus □ Sektion: ja □ nein □

Weitere Bemerkungen (z. B. Todesursache):

► Das Beilegen des Arztbriefes und/oder des Krankenhausentlassungsbriefes ist in Fällen schwerer UAW hilfreich. ◄

Wer wurde zusätzlich informiert: BfArM □   Hersteller □   PEI □   Sonstige:

Name des Arztes: Klinik: ja □ nein □ (ggf. Stempel)   Datum:

Fachrichtung:

Anschrift:
                                                                    _____
Telefon-Nr.:   Unterschrift

Figure 8. AkdÄ reporting form, contemporary.
(⟨http://www.akdae.de/50/50/05UAWBerichtsbogen.pdf⟩)

forms, German doctors are granted space for additional comments. They are also asked to check off whether they have reported the reaction to the BGA, the manufacturer, or AkdÄ. Each of these organizations promulgates the same form, though they place their own names on the letterhead.

The *Stufenplan* offers a multi-stage process to negotiate which, if any, cases deserve policy interventions. During a minimum of two annual meetings, representatives from state health ministries, AkdÄ, the drug manufacturers association, and the Federal Health Office discuss new case reports. If officials at BfArM—the 1994 successor institute to the BGA—suspect something is amiss, they can initiate a formal exchange of case reports. According to the law, this Risk Level I (*Gefahrenstufe I*) is intended to generate data on the frequency with which cases have occurred, suggest possible causes, and indicate dangers to public health.[60] BfArM can then call a special meeting, thereby initiating Risk Level II (*Gefahrenstufe II*). At this stage, the manufacturer can defend their drug, and other medical experts can present their findings about the adverse reaction events. Health officials then can decide to commission further research, require changes to the dosage or treatment regimen, or even recall a drug from the market.[61]

While the *Stufenplan* originally called for open meetings and public announcements of decisions, few face-to-face meetings took place during the 1990s. Instead, the process shifted to written correspondence, e-mail, and telephone conversations. According to an AkdÄ assessment, of seventy-eight cases in 1994 and fifty-two cases in 1995 that reached Risk Level II, none resulted in actual meetings.[62] In an effort to promote greater public attention to drug risks, AkdÄ then started to publish not only official warnings, but also *Stufenplan* correspondence in the weekly medical journal, *Deutsches Ärzteblatt*. As a result, interim findings of otherwise closed proceedings were made available to practicing physicians across Germany.

AkdÄ as a Quasi-Public Organization

The decision to inform physicians and the public about ongoing proceedings was challenged in a 1995 court case. Cordichin, a combination of Chinidin (a treatment for heart arrhythmia) and Verapamil (a calcium channel blocker), was used to treat heart conditions starting in 1970.[63] Some twenty years later, reports to the Drug Commission indicated that the drug was causing ventricular fibrillation, cardiac arrest, and ventricular tachycardia, a potentially fatal irregularity in the normal heart rhythm. In a seemingly paradoxical development, instead of stabilizing heart rhythms, the drug instead increased the frequency with which arrhythmic spasms occurred. AkdÄ published a notice about the drug in mid-1991, and suggested that physicians switch to alternative treatments.[64] The commission also asked doctors to look out for adverse reactions to Cordichin among their patients.

After AkdÄ collected reports and shared them with BfArM officials, the government initiated Risk Level I of the *Stufenplan* with a letter to the manufacturer, Minden Pharma.[65] Minden, a small division of the larger pharmaceutical company Knoll, had to answer a series of questions about the drug, document cases of adverse reactions worldwide, provide production figures, list countries where the drug had been reviewed by regulatory agencies, and provide a commentary on the drug's therapeutic significance compared to alternative treatments. Well over a year later, BfArM initiated Risk Level II, arguing that the increased risks from Cordichin were unjustifiable in light of the ready availability of alternative therapies.[66] In their communication with the company, health officials offered the company four weeks to defend their drug.

AkdÄ then planned to again warn physicians about Cordichin in an article containing excerpts from the BfArM letter. Knoll sued, arguing that the article impinged on the company's still-valid market authorization. An administrative court in Köln soon agreed, and blocked AkdÄ from publishing BfArM statements, its own assessment of the drug, or warnings to physicians.[67] The court also punished the commission by awarding the company DM 500,000 in compensation. Upon appeal, the case went to the superior administrative court for the state Nordrhein-Westfalen, which agreed with the decision of the lower court.[68] In both decisions, justices considered AkdÄ's decision to distribute material from *Stufenplan* correspondence a "premature publication of preliminary risk assessments."[69] More generally, the courts criticized the state-like structure and authority AkdÄ had assumed since the 1950s.

Judges found fault with AkdÄ's stance as a quasi-public institution and wanted to differentiate its role as a member in the *Stufenplan* from its role as an advisory body to the medical profession. Accordingly, in order for AkdÄ to participate in the *Stufenplan*, it had to follow guidelines that allowed companies to defend their medicines in private meetings. As a legal commentator sympathetic to Knoll wrote, "The interests of public health do not reach so far as to justify an intervention in the market."[70] Likewise, the courts feared that published warnings about side effects would drive the drug from the market before safety tests were completed. In the eyes of the German legal system, AkdÄ should choose between its private role, guaranteeing its right to publish opinions and analysis, and its public role, under which it could only make restricted claims.

In response, AkdÄ argued that its ability to maintain authority over prescribing practices would be undermined if it had to wait for BfArM to publish warnings about dangerous drugs. Its leaders also invoked the protection of patients as their primary mandate. Thus AkdÄ's director Bruno Müller-

Oerlinghausen argued vehemently that any interference with the organization would promote manufacturers' short-term financial interests to the detriment of public health.[71] Fearing a public backlash, the government agreed in 1996 to formally recognize AkdÄ's right to publish warnings through a revision to the Drug Law.[72] Changes to the law in 1998, however, failed to grant AkdÄ permission to report about ongoing *Stufenplan* proceedings.[73] The commission must instead wait for BfArM to issue a final ruling before warning physicians or recommending changes in prescriptions.

Maintaining Guild Control

In the period between 1970 and the present, the Drug Commission first consolidated its position and then lost ground as the BGA and BfArM gradually asserted authority over adverse drug reactions. In a critical development, AkdÄ's ability to inform practicing physicians about drug risks was challenged when German courts held that the commission had to choose either to act as a government agency or serve as an external advisory board. Since that time, AkdÄ position papers and press statements have articulated its desire to remain in the network of organizations that oversee side effects, while retaining its historical independence from industry and the government. Above all else, officials want to provide physicians with information about prescription drugs independent of the pharmaceutical industry. Despite the legal challenges posed by the Cordichin case, AkdÄ officials have succeeded in maintaining their status both in the *Stufenplan* and as a key site for collecting reports of adverse reactions. The organization thus engages in three complementary activities: collecting reports of adverse reactions, collaborating with the federal government in the *Stufenplan*, and informing physicians which drugs they should or should not prescribe to patients.

AkdÄ's role in the network of organizations that address side effects in Germany relies on a construction of the patient as an individual who needs professional advice and protection from industry and the state. Cases ranging from thalidomide to Cordichin were used to expand professional authority over drug testing in Germany, not to mobilize greater state regulation. AkdÄ also argues that these cases illustrate the need for the medical profession to protect the public after drugs are marketed. Unlike in the United States, this construction of the patient was only rarely contested and underwent few changes in recent decades. Patients themselves have figured far less prominently in the social structuring of authority over adverse reactions in Germany than in the United States. This parallels their comparative absence from debates over drug laws and procedures for clinical trials. The network of organizations that collect, compare, and respond to side effects in Germany shields members from some of the political demands and concerns about transparency found in the United States. Above all else, it has prevented competing constructions of the patient from becoming a driver of policy change.

Pharmaceutical Consumers as Test Subjects

Very different institutions in the United States and Germany mediate the translation of side effects from individual, unwanted, physical and / or psychological drug reactions to data sets used in policy decisions. Unlike subjects participating in clinical trials, patients are rarely warned that they, in effect, are taking part in an experiment when using prescription drugs. Though rarely considered a formal test, professional associations, government regulatory agencies, and pharmaceutical companies monitor real-world therapy. Standardized reporting forms and formal routines for information exchange and review have transformed the open market to serve as an extension of the clinical trial. Testing thus continues beyond the confines of the clinical setting and includes far more diverse populations once drugs are marketed.

In the United States, the FDA has historically preferred to rely on premarket testing to determine drug safety and efficacy. Clinical trials offered government regulators greater control over physicians and patients than postmarket evaluation. Once drugs were approved, the agency faced technical challenges related to standardizing and comparing reports, as well as political risks from adverse publicity. As a solution to this dilemma, FDA officials sought to tightly circumscribe the arena for quantitative postmarket evaluations while remaining open to some "spontaneous" qualitative reporting. In Germany, the stronger self-regulatory position of the medical profession prevented the construction of a stark division between test and market. AkdÄ could employ qualitative review methods both inside and outside the clinical setting. Observation of patients thus proceeded with less attention to formal methods of double-blinding and clinical controls.

Successful postmarket data collection, like premarket clinical trials, relies on physicians and patients to follow prescribed social norms. Each of the institutions described here tried to structure the doctor-patient relationship to produce objective and interpretable reports about drugs outside of the controlled clinical setting. In both countries, government authorities and the medical profession expected patients to recognize adverse reactions, assist physicians in reporting them to central authorities, and then continue to take other prescription drugs. However difficult it may be to discipline patients to report adverse reactions, physicians too must be trained to complete and submit forms. A standardized product requires a standardized producer. Authorities thus sought to convince physicians to complete reports in a timely manner using fixed criteria to evaluate and record side effects.

Contrasts between the two countries' therapeutic cultures delineated illness and narrowed treatment options, determined social roles for patients and physicians, and shaped the organizations that governed the pharmaceutical market. Local negotiations over drug safety and medicinal risks ultimately determined the methods used to collect, compare, and respond to adverse reactions. In these ways, organizations—including the AMA and FDA in the United States and AkdÄ and BfArM in Germany—followed strategies for risk management that fit with each country's therapeutic culture.

Between 1950 and the present, different constructions of "the patient" in the two countries led to marked contrasts between the organizations that sought to manage drug risks. In the United States, the AMA lost its regulatory role once the FDA asserted significant authority in this area. As a professional association, the AMA could shape practitioners' norms and set standards for drug safety and efficacy. The Council on Drugs positioned itself between industry and ill people, promising to protect naïve patients from dangerous medicines. It nevertheless failed to assemble the financial and scientific resources necessary to build a large database for adverse reactions and could not intervene to force drug withdrawals. In contrast, the FDA built databases from hospital reports in an effort to generate more precise causal links between drugs and adverse reactions. Regulatory action in the United States depended on statistical proof of harm to patients. In parallel with more rapid drug approvals by the mid-1980s that responded to activists and reflected a consumer-based definition of the patient, the FDA turned to physicians in private practices and individual patients as data sources.

In Germany, a network of organizations regulated the pharmaceutical market. As a professional association, AkdÄ had the authority and legitimacy to convince physicians of the necessity for reporting adverse reactions. It could then promote a construction of the patient as a German citizen who needed professional guidance and oversight. In addition, consensus among experts from AkdÄ, BfArM, and the pharmaceutical industry prevented the emergence of debates about data standardization and methods for determining drug safety. In cases of drug withdrawals due to adverse reactions, the network suffered comparatively little political damage, and procedures for risk review underwent only minor changes. More recently, European regulatory harmonization and centralization increased the German government's role in adverse reactions. Nevertheless, AkdÄ has positioned itself as the key representative of the patient in regulatory discussions. It also holds a carefully managed monopoly of the expertise needed to analyze drug risks.

Systems for recording and responding to adverse reactions are tied to political structures for expert engagement. Because of differences in their therapeutic cultures, Germany has vested political and regulatory authority in the medical profession, while the United States has adopted a state-centered approach. The relative ability of patient groups to organize and demand access to clinical trials, observe and participate in regulatory decision making, and reshape boundaries of postmarketing data collection consequently differ in these two countries. These differences have serious implications for current and future approaches to drug regulation, the subject of the concluding chapter.

6 Conclusion

International Harmonization and the Future of Drug Regulation

DIFFERENCES IN DRUG REGULATION BETWEEN THE United States and Germany since the early 1950s are readily apparent in drug laws, clinical trials, and postmarketing surveillance. What should today's international travelers and tomorrow's global citizens make of the contrasts? Are they merely quaint reminders of twentieth-century regulatory styles and medical norms that will · soon be displaced by global regimes? Therapeutic cultures, as we have seen, are the product of ongoing negotiations among the state, the medical profession, industry, and disease-based organizations. While they are regularly in flux, certain key features have held constant for each country between 1950 and the present (Table 6). As a result, even though the international harmonization of therapeutic cultures may appear inevitable, they retain specific national characteristics that will resist globalization.

As discussed in the introduction, pharmaceuticals play an expanding role in the areas of international trade, intellectual property, and health security. Pharmaceuticals are also integral to contemporary discussions about national sovereignty and human rights. Illustrative of the degree to which drugs and drug companies have

TABLE 6 / THERAPEUTIC CULTURES

United States	Germany
Direct citizen ↔ state relations	Medical profession mediates relations between the public and the state
Physicians serve as individual experts	Physicians organized as a communal profession/guild
Regulatory authority concentrated in the state	Regulatory authority shared across a network of the state, industry, and the medical profession
Quantitative testing methods are imposed by the FDA	Qualitative testing methods arise from communal norms and self-imposed standards

captured widespread attention, the novelist John Le Carré's most recent pro-
tagonist, unlike the spies working for Cold War–era nations in so many of his
previous novels, travels the globe to expose a corporate cover-up of failed drug
trials in Africa. When he confronts a British civil servant with his responsibility
for cracking down on an offending company, the latter responds, "You think
countries run the fucking world? It's 'God save our multinational' they're
singing these days."[1]

   In a case of reality mimicking fiction, thirty Nigerian families sued Pfizer in
U.S. federal court shortly after Le Carré's novel appeared, claiming that the
pharmaceutical firm had conducted an unethical clinical trial on their children.[2] Coupled to a decline in the ability of national regulatory bodies and
legal institutions to control multinational firms, other groups—notably non-
governmental organizations—have stepped into a watchdog role. The expansion of multinational firms is also coupled to greater bi-directional information
flow with people in developing countries. Their growth has also fueled the
formation of global governance bodies and the willingness to at least entertain
international lawsuits in federal courts. The suit against Pfizer illustrates that
clinical trials must meet stringent ethical norms, even when held in seemingly
remote areas. Corporate sponsors can be held accountable if physicians—
including those operating in therapeutic settings distant from the United
States—fail to meet these norms.[3]

   Very similar issues of medical ethics and professional norms are now pos-
ing challenges to therapeutic cultures around the globe. The vocabulary and
terms of negotiations among the principal actors in medical policy and politics
thus are taking on an increasingly universal appearance. Nevertheless, national
therapeutic cultures remain active and politically salient at the start of the

twenty-first century. This concluding chapter first reviews key findings about drug laws, clinical trials, and postmarket surveillance in the United States and Germany. Next, we explore international harmonization as an emerging fourth arena in which variation among therapeutic cultures will play a major role. The chapter closes with some thoughts on the future of drug regulation and governance in a system of distributed power.

The Patient in the United States and Germany

Striking contrasts are apparent between the United States and Germany, despite important similarities in the two countries. The concept of therapeutic cultures helps explain how different constructions of "the patient" at play in a network of key actors in medical policy and politics ultimately shaped drug regulation (Table 7). Therapeutic cultures shaped political negotiations on drug laws, medical debates over testing methods, and techniques used to oversee drugs on the market. In each country, negotiations over medical issues of drug safety and efficacy are coupled to broader concerns about the distribution of power and public representation. While the major actors in the arena of drug regulation are very similar in the two countries, they relate to one another in very different ways. In the United States, the primary nexus of power is between the state and citizens, whereas in Germany, regulatory control is distributed across a formal network of actors. This contrast fuels differences in testing methods and approaches to postmarket surveillance.

During the second half of the twentieth century, medicine became a site for debates over the role of experts, professionals, and the patient. As a result, medical policy now involves mobilization of actors above and beyond the medical profession. Likewise, controversies regarding drug safety and patient rights occur in settings above and beyond the clinical trial. As we have seen, the process of regulatory rule-making and enforcement, clinical testing, and market surveillance are three important sites for the influence of therapeutic cultures.

In the first of these sites, described in Chapter 2, the U.S. Congress increased the FDA's authority and mandated formal rules for drug evaluation in response to precipitating events, notably cases of widespread adverse drug reactions. Congress and the FDA expected government control over premarket testing to protect patients otherwise open to abuses by industry and the medical profession. By virtue of its centralization in the FDA, drug regulation became very politicized in the United States, with competing social actors demanding weaker or stronger restrictions on new pharmaceuticals. Drug regulation also evolved into a site for patients and disease-based organizations to articulate their opposition to government paternalism.

TABLE 7 / "THE PATIENT"

Years	United States	Germany
1930s–1960s	"Misled" public deserves more information about the content of medicines, mediated by the medical profession	Under the Nazis, patients are bodies that should suffer in parallel with the war effort; after WWII, autonomous patients deserve care and individual attention by the medical profession
1960s–1980s	"Guinea pigs" need state protection from industry and the medical profession	"Frightened" public needs reassurance and protection by the medical profession, industry, and government
1980s–2000	Active and self-aware consumers participate in every stage of health care decision making	All but invisible to politics and health policy, where attention is focused on costs and the division of authority among government, industry, and the medical profession

Drug regulation in Germany, by contrast, occasioned fewer conflicts among industry, the medical profession, and the government. The principal actors in medical policy did not offer alternative constructions of "the patient" in order to expand their control over drug testing. Absent a specific decision-making agency or precise regulatory moment, patients did not mobilize to demand speedier pharmaceutical approvals or to bring about changes in testing methods.

Clinical trials are crucial to the production of knowledge about a drug's effects on humans. In this second site for therapeutic cultures, the United States centralized a quest for objective drug assessment under FDA control. This agency demanded multiple controlled clinical trials and statistical evaluation of their results before approving medicines. Drug testing in Germany, on the other hand, remained under the exclusive control of the medical profession. Physicians testing medicines in Germany relied primarily on qualitative methods to assess how patients reacted to new drugs. Since German physicians had greater control over drug testing in the clinical setting than their American counterparts, statisticians made few inroads into the clinical trial.

Case studies of Terramycin, thalidomide, propranolol, interleukin-2, and indinavir in Chapters 3 and 4 illustrate important changes between 1950 and the present in each country. In the United States, the FDA used its regulatory authority to force changes in the clinical setting and to establish norms for doctor-patient relations. In Germany, changes in testing methods were gradual and arose from within the medical profession. Reports of drug tests remained largely internal to the medical community. By the end of the twentieth century, patients in the United States challenged the status quo of medical politics and promoted changes to testing methods and regulatory approaches. In Germany, fewer changes took place. The medical profession largely retained its authority to speak for "the patient," even as the setting for medical policy and politics shifted to the European Union.

Different constructions of "the patient" in the two countries led to marked contrasts between the organizations that sought to monitor approved medicines, the subject of Chapter 5. In the United States, the AMA lost its regulatory role once the FDA asserted significant authority in this area. As a professional association, the AMA could shape practitioners' norms and set standards for drug safety and efficacy. Its Council on Drugs positioned itself between industry and ill people, promising to protect naïve patients from dangerous medicines. Physicians nevertheless failed to assemble the financial and scientific resources necessary to build a large database for adverse reactions and could not intervene to force drug withdrawals. In contrast, the FDA built databases from hospital reports in order to generate causal links between drugs and adverse reactions. In parallel with more rapid drug approvals by the mid-1980s that responded to activists and reflected a consumer-based definition of the patient, the FDA turned to physicians in private practices and even individual patients as data sources.

In Germany, a network of organizations regulated the pharmaceutical market. As a professional association, the Drug Commission had the authority and legitimacy to convince physicians to report adverse reactions. It could then promote a construction of the patient as a German citizen who needed professional guidance and oversight. In addition, consensus among experts from the medical profession, the federal government, and the pharmaceutical industry prevented the emergence of public debates and scandals about drug safety. In cases of drug withdrawals due to adverse reactions, the network suffered comparatively little political damage, and procedures for risk review underwent only minor changes. More recently, European regulatory harmonization and centralization have actually served to increase the government's role in adverse reactions. Nevertheless, the Drug Commission has positioned itself as the sole representative of the patient in regulatory discussions while judiciously cultivating the expertise needed to analyze drug risks.

Medicine and the State in the Two Therapeutic Cultures

It has become fashionable in recent years to discuss the "crisis in governance" and simultaneous "breakdown in civil society" currently afflicting advanced industrialized nations.[4] This study suggests that both governing institutions and civil society are alive and well at the start of the twenty-first century. The loci for political action, citizen mobilization, and governance have changed. From an exclusive focus on global and national politics, we as analysts must turn to the doctor-patient relationship and interactions between citizens and regulatory agencies to understand contemporary public life. Activities in these sites create the environment in which the state, industry, professions, and non-governmental organizations interact to formulate policy.

Ongoing innovation in regulatory policy in the United States, as we have seen, is made necessary by awareness of deficits in the health care system and mobilization of actors in the therapeutic culture. The existence of analogous deficits is less politically salient in Germany, since the medical profession largely speaks for the patient. Furthermore, the less stringently enforced boundary between testing and market historically has made medicines available to patients sooner than in the United States. The very need for Americans to take an active role in learning about their ailments and the near necessity of confronting physicians and government officials is evidence of a health care system under extreme stress. Often lauded as a positive outcome of a more transparent and open political process, patient mobilization also offers evidence of the failure of American health care to respond to citizen needs, in contrast to the German system.

From the observation and control of patients by physicians and the state, a multilateral system of surveillance has emerged with state and professional authorities disciplined by public demands for oversight, transparency, and participation in decision making. Indeed, mutual observation and surveillance among individuals and institutions form a cornerstone of contemporary democracies. Upon moving the capital from Bonn to Berlin, the German government intentionally selected architects who would design buildings that allow for two-way observation of democracy at work. A glass tower on top of the renovated Reichstag, now seat of the German Bundestag, is designed so that parliamentary representatives can see visitors walking around above them as they debate issues of public policy. Citing Germany's dark historical precedents, the principal architect argues, "Grand politics is not possible without grand architecture." In an effort to influence the future of German politics, he and his colleagues designed "institutional transparency" into the architecture of the new German capital.[5]

Transparency and public display also play a role in maintaining public confidence in health authorities. National therapeutic cultures thus remain politically salient at the start of the twenty-first century. Approaches used to generate medical knowledge and verify the efficacy of treatments have been transformed in modern Western societies from networks of personal trust and familiarity to impersonal systems and institutions. As the historian Steven

Shapin explains, "The modern place of knowledge here appears not a gentleman's drawing room but as a great Panopticon of Truth."[6] The roles of trust and personal trustworthiness that he identifies as crucial to establishing scientific truths have not been displaced by new impersonal regimes of quantification and bureaucratic control. Germany has retained the personal touch of the physician to mediate between citizens and institutions that certify the safety and efficacy of drugs. The United States has made political accommodation for citizens to themselves gain the expertise and authority to oversee and interact with "impersonal" knowledge production. The contrast between these two therapeutic cultures' loci for creating trust in medicine and medical care is particularly important in light of an emerging regime for international regulatory harmonization.

The Patient in an International Regime

Over the course of the last decade, European, American, and Japanese regulatory agencies and drug manufacturers have worked closely to create harmonized procedures for the global introduction of new drugs. In a series of meetings formally known as the "International Conference on Harmonisation of Technical Requirements for Registration of Pharmaceuticals for Human Use" (ICH), invited members have gathered to discuss methods for standardizing pre-clinical and clinical testing as well as procedures for regulatory review. ICH began in 1990 with a jointly sponsored meeting of the European Commission, European Federation of Pharmaceutical Industries and Associations, FDA, Pharmaceutical Research and Manufacturers of America, Japan's Ministry of Health, Labor and Welfare, and Japan Pharmaceutical Manufacturers Association. The name ICH is more closely associated with the process of harmonization than the actual conferences, of which five have been held as of spring 2003, with a sixth scheduled for fall 2003.

ICH's primary purpose is to harmonize technical guidelines and requirements for medicinal drug registrations. The industry and regulators have found their interests converging over the last decade with a mutual desire to reduce the use of "human, animal, and material resources" as they work to "eliminate unnecessary delay in the global development and registration of new drugs."[7] Since clinical trials now consume over half of drug companies' R&D spending, manufacturers are highly motivated to cut down on the quantity and variety of tests required by national regulatory agencies. As described in Chapters 3 and 4, criticisms have long been levied against the FDA for taking too long to review and approve drugs. In recent years, these criticisms have expanded to include some regulatory agencies in European countries and even the newly formed European Agency for the Evaluation of Medicinal Products (EMEA).[8]

The long-term goal of ICH, however, is far more ambitious than to simply rationalize drug approvals. Participants intend to overcome obstacles created by different medical and cultural traditions and to create a world in which only one set of research trials is performed before the global marketing of a new drug can take place. In their vision of the future, data produced in this now-crucial experiment (or centrally coordinated set of clinical trials) will be reviewed using uniform standards. Recognizing the near-impossibility of dismantling well-established regulatory agencies, ICH hopes nonetheless that uniform product submissions will lead to the same conclusions regarding a drug's "approvability" around the world. Reflecting on a decade of work in 2000, ICH proudly announced that it has been "successful in achieving harmonization, initially of technical guidelines and more recently on the format and content of registration applications."[9] ICH leaders expect that pharmaceutical companies will soon be able to submit a single electronic dossier on a new drug to regulatory agencies in the United States, European Union, and Japan.[10]

ICH participants appreciate the complexities associated with this goal and do not advocate making the move to complete regulatory harmonization in a single step. Instead, the organization is approaching harmonization incrementally, moving tentatively from toxicology and pharmacology standards to the more complex political and social issues that arise from human clinical tests and postmarket studies. Harmonization proceeds incrementally from technical discussions in "expert working groups" to consultation with affiliated organizations. "Consensus drafts" from the working groups are reviewed by the regulatory agencies, and scientific experts outside the ICH group are asked to assess specific proposals for their impact on drug quality, safety, and efficacy.[11]

Once the industry and regulators have reached agreement, new standards are implemented through domestic regulations and regional procedures.[12] ICH thus does not have the goal of supplanting regulatory agencies like the FDA or EMEA. Topics discussed in the different working groups range over the entire terrain of drug testing from pharmacokinetics to clinical trials. In addition, working groups have moved beyond the bounded space of clinical trials when discussing new modes of communication among regulatory agencies. These include sharing information about adverse reactions and, more broadly, on regulatory approaches. Well over forty guidelines and standards are in various stages of the ICH process. Consensus was reached quickly in the areas of drug quality standards, necessary toxicity tests, and expectations for good clinical practice.[13] Clinical trials and postmarket surveillance have proven more difficult to harmonize.

The ICH process reflects lessons learned from the long and at times bitter discussions leading to the opening of EMEA in 1996. Both ICH and EMEA do more than find common ground for agreement on technical safety standards.

Harmonization of standards assumes both that social systems should be steered in a particular direction and that an institution for risk assessment and control can be built through the mutual recognition of techniques and technologies in the clinic.[14] Unifying risk perceptions by physicians in charge of clinical trials and adverse reaction reporting will likely prove a Herculean task. As the historical cases presented throughout this book suggest, medicine—especially when asked to identify and measure risks posed by innovative drugs—has distinctive cultural traits. It is difficult to imagine that a "voluntary" process can force a globally standardized regime onto doctors and patients in the constrained environment of clinical trials, much less in the broader environment of regular medical care.

Yet, unlike the standardization of pre-clinical and clinical testing in the United States that depended on the FDA's regulatory apparatus of surveillance and formal rules, ICH is seeking to harmonize drug testing through protocols and voluntary agreement. As I have argued, drug testing is intimately linked to broader conceptions of how physicians, regulatory agencies, drug companies, and patients should interact. In this regard, ICH has the potential to improve medical care by finding an appropriate balance among competing regulatory styles. As a consensual regulatory streamlining process, it will also have great impact on clinical trials and ultimately on medical practice and the authority of experts in Europe, the United States, and elsewhere. It need not function, as some critics have argued, to lessen regulatory oversight and reduce protections for patients.[15]

At the same time, this process for international harmonization assumes that national health politics, political or medical representation of different populations, and issues of ethics and equity are irrelevant to drug safety and efficacy. Attention to therapeutic cultures reveals that scientific and medical testing are themselves important sites for politics in the United States. Testing is less politicized in Germany, but only because the medical profession has maintained certain forms of guild authority and "pre-modern" relationships of trust. Nevertheless, the recent emergence of citizen initiatives related to biotechnology and success of the Green Party indicate that established parties and interest groups are failing to meet citizen demands.[16]

Contrasts between these two therapeutic cultures suggest that enacting international regulatory harmonization will face potentially serious criticisms. On one front, patient activists will challenge a technocratic system that excludes their concerns. From another front, physicians will challenge a standardized regime that reduces their professional expertise. In effect, by assuming that patients can be constructed as nothing more than data sources, and physicians as little more than data gatherers, ICH participants are leaving themselves vulnerable to attacks from at least two sides. How they respond and adapt to expectations for participatory democracy from constituents in very different political and cultural settings will determine the success of this venture.

Evolving Systems of Governance and the Future of Drug Regulation

Medical clinics often function as microcosms of democratic states, dealing with the same issues of representation, equity, innovation, data gathering and distribution, and appropriateness of decision-making procedures as are found on a larger, overtly political scale. Disease-based organizations now argue, in essence, that if countries get their medical systems right, they will get their democratic politics right. This feature is strongly at play in debates over the role of pharmaceutical companies in international trade and demands for strong ethical standards in clinical trials. Public involvement in regulatory decisions differs in important ways among even similarly advanced industrialized democracies. Nevertheless, aspects of medical politics once localized to individual nations, including definitions of drug safety and efficacy, standards for clinical trials, and methods for observing patient ↔ drug interactions, now play out at an international level as well.

The authority to govern, that is, to set standards, as well as to define relations between physicians and patients and to enact and enforce rules, derives as much from the ability to classify and characterize people as it does from the ability to order human relations. This authority is no longer situated solely in the state or medical profession, but instead is spread across a network of actors. Comparative studies of risk and regulation are often based on contrasts among clearly delineated states. For this reason, categories such as power, legitimacy, and democracy are tied to traditional notions of the state. In future studies of international regulatory harmonization, we have the opportunity to problematize existing rigid definitions of "the state."

As we have seen, contemporary states are made up of a complex ensemble of actors and institutions that negotiate issues such as drug regulation using cultural resources unique to each country. One means by which agencies responsible for consumer health and safety can hope to harmonize these ensembles is through transparent negotiations that make institutions responsive to civic expectations. At the same time, transparency in Europe and North America is based on culturally conditioned ways of seeing the state and "seeing like a state."[17] Risk assessment in drug regulation therefore is more than a process of deciding trade-offs between safe and dangerous drugs. It is connected to aspects of public involvement, democratic representation, and modes of organizing the state and civil society at the start of the twenty-first century.

Drug regulation as practiced in the United States and, to a lesser extent, in Germany is an exercise in extreme reductionism. Decisions granting market approvals are built upon the effort to test a single compound against a single disease, despite enormous variation among patients, diseases, and states of health or illness. Likewise, safety and efficacy have been defined either as easily measured biological responses to drugs or in terms of their economic costs and benefits. This reductionist approach also lies behind the effort to design patient-specific treatments based on genetic profiles. While promising treatments customized to individuals, "personalized medicine" will likely involve direct negotiations about privacy and ownership of genetic data between individuals and corporations.[18] More generally, the evidence presented here documents the need for a more complex understanding of risk and regulation that accounts for and incorporates a greater number of political players and perspectives on what it means to treat disease with pharmaceutical drugs.

Similarly, creating a pinnacle of experts to carry out international harmonization may work in the short run, but its long-term success will derive only from a broader base of legitimacy that incorporates concerns from other quarters. This will almost certainly require greater attention to issues of drug prices and availability of health care to patients in developing countries and in poorer populations of industrialized nations. These features were carefully excluded from twentieth century regulatory policies aimed at defining drug safety and efficacy. They will nevertheless dominate future policy making in this area.

Foreshadowing a debate over drug prices that may sharply influence future innovation, clinical testing, and regulation, several reports in the past year have claimed radically different costs borne by the industry for drug development. A study by Joseph DiMasi of the Tufts Center for the Study of Drug Development found that a new drug's development requires an average outlay of $402 million over the course of ten to fifteen years.[19] With the addition of an "opportunity cost of capital" of $400 million, DiMasi argues that it takes over $800 million to bring a new drug from the laboratory to patients. Pharmaceutical manufacturers have seized upon this figure to defend pricing policies that are increasingly scrutinized by the press, politicians, and general public. At the same time, the Ralph Nader–affiliated nonprofit organization, Public Citizen, contests these sums. Its Health Research Group has presented evidence that once research support from the National Institutes of Health (NIH) and federal tax breaks are taken into account, the cost is closer to $150 million for new chemical entities and between $71 million and $118 million for all drugs brought to market.[20] Other groups have presented evidence that the industry spends more on marketing, advertising, and administration than on R&D, thereby profiting from disease while employing "public interest" rhetoric to avoid greater government oversight.[21] Drug cost is another dimension of health care that individual patients must increasingly understand in order to choose among therapeutic options.

Yet medical politics are not parsed out into separate debates about drug prices, innovation, clinical testing methods, or regulatory decisions. Instead, the key issues today and in years to come involve the politics of identity. Regulation is an important locus for patients to identify and create their identities. In the United States, disease-based organizations have adopted a strategy of visual presentation of patients' ailments and direct political confrontation with government authorities. The comparison with Germany presented here shows that this is a very American strategy of connecting the "invisible" world of disease to the "visible" world of government decision making. In turn, the government is pushed to fund medical research and deploy risk assessment procedures as instrumental modes of political accommodation. American politics consequently retains a remarkably utopian vision as patients, physicians, companies, and regulatory agencies articulate different hopeful versions of the future.[22]

In Germany and in the emerging European Union, by contrast, elite scientific and expert modes of visualization are inscribed into the practices of political institutions. As a result, political consensus dominates and transparency is oriented to the decision-making process, rather than its content. The principal actors in medical policy are far more concerned with pragmatic realities than utopian political visions. In the emerging ICH regime, attention to individual risk trade-offs will likely feature less prominently. Instead, political debates and policy initiatives will need to connect visible features of drug regulation with less visible aspects of political risks to government agencies and international regimes, along with patients' concerns regarding equity and the availability of medicines.

Nearly twenty years ago, the medical expert M. N. G. Dukes asked, "Has it ever struck you that, for some of us who live in the world of drug therapy, a medicine so very easily becomes more important—certainly more central and more tangible—than the hundreds of thousands of people who take it? It has a name, protected by law and patent, whilst its users are but a gray, anonymous, heterogeneous mass."[23] Disease-based organizations and the policy changes they promoted in the United States have elevated the "gray mass" of users in many ways. In a different political context, the political standing of the German medical profession prevented patients from being treated as a "mass."

Looking to the future, only policies that promote the tangible expression of patients' perspectives and give them a voice and a visible presence in decision making will lead to success in the international harmonization of drug regulation. The challenge ahead is to design working institutions for a polity of unprecedented size and diversity. Only if we rise to that challenge by incorporating multiple voices and designing transparent decision-making procedures—ones that grant visibility and participation to patients—will globalization become something more than the reduction of trade barriers that benefits a minority of the population in advanced industrialized countries.

Appendix

Research Methods and Case Study Selection

This project is grounded in methods of qualitative research common to the social sciences. Much of the analysis is based on a careful reading of published documents, including articles from scientific and medical journals, congressional hearings, policy documents, newspaper accounts, secondary sources, and materials posted on Internet web sites. These sources are roughly parallel for the two countries. Unsurprisingly, there were some asymmetries in the primary source materials. In the United States, I obtained a great deal of information directly from the FDA through Freedom of Information Act filings. This gave me access to several complete New Drug Applications, transcripts from some advisory committee hearings, and detailed correspondence between the FDA and manufacturers. I supplemented these sources with archival research at the National Library of Medicine and the American Institute for the History of Pharmacy, both of which have holdings on the medical profession, pharmaceuticals, and the pharmaceutical industry. In Germany, I obtained information for the period up to the mid-1960s from the National Archives (in Germany, as in most other European countries, government documents less than thirty years old typically are not available for research use) and also gathered materials from the Federal Chamber of Physicians, the pharmaceutical industry trade association, and from holdings at drug companies.

During research trips in the United States and Germany, I enhanced these materials with semi-structured interviews. Questions were prepared in advance; however, I intentionally structured interviews to allow follow-up queries to insightful responses. While a valuable "primary" source by themselves, the interviews were also very helpful for gaining access to private archives and document centers otherwise not open to the public.

Case Study Selection

Clinical trials lie at the center of this book, both figuratively and literally. From an early stage in my research, I focused on clinical testing and sought out materials on specific drugs that had been tested and reviewed by regulatory authorities in both countries. The pharmaceuticals I chose for more careful research map onto the five decades between 1950 and 2000. Case studies examine Terramycin (an antibiotic), thalidomide (an anti-depressant), propranolol (a heart medication), interleukin-2 (an anticancer drug), and indinavir (an AIDS medication). Cases were selected to highlight differences between medicines with close association to the cultural and historical changes that took place in clinical testing during the latter half of the twentieth century. I applied the same selection criteria in both countries to avoid incommensurable data sets.

First, I looked for drugs that were primarily developed, tested, and marketed by the private sector. Federally funded organizations such as the U.S. National Institutes of Health do develop and transfer medicines to the private sector. Their testing protocols, however, face fewer questions about industry influence and improper patient recruitment than are of interest here.

Second, each drug was explicitly not the first available treatment for the intended condition. Regulatory agencies, expert advisers, and practicing physicians understandably feel special pressure to approve a drug quickly when it is the only treatment available for a medical condition. As we have seen, the degree of pressure exerted on government regulators to approve drugs quickly underwent important changes in the time period I describe. At the same time, pharmaceutical companies learned to narrow medical conditions and describe therapies in such a way that almost every new drug now appears to treat a unique condition.

Third, I sought out medicines that were intended to treat diseases affecting large populations in both countries. Although some ended up with a limited market in their final use, during clinical trials each was thought to offer a therapeutic advance that would guarantee a major market for the drug company. This feature ensures that the manufacturer was sufficiently motivated to stick with the drug, even when challenged on its safety or efficacy by either the American or the German regulatory system.

Finally, the cases intentionally offer an approximate chronology of the main foci of medical attention during the latter half of the twentieth century: infectious disease, anxiety / sleeplessness, heart disease, cancer, and AIDS.

Notes

Abbreviations

AkdÄ   Arzneimittelkommission der deutschen Ärzteschaft, Köln, Germany
Boehringer   Boehringer Ingelheim GmbH, Firmen- und Familienarchiv, Ingelheim,
                Germany; documents provided courtesy of Ruth Linck
Bundesarchiv   Federal Republic of Germany, National Archives, Koblenz, Germany
FDA Files   U.S. Government, Department of Health and Human Services, Food and Drug
                Administration, History Office, Rockville, Md.
IGM   Institut für Geschichte der Medizin der Freien Universität Berlin, Berlin,
                Germany
NLM   National Library of Medicine, Bethesda, Md.

Chapter One

1. DiMasi, "Economics of Pharmaceutical Innovation"; see also DiMasi, "New Drug Innovation"; Pharmaceutical Research and Manufacturers of America, *Why Do Prescription Drugs Cost So Much?*; for a significantly lower estimate of drug development costs, see Young and Surrusco, *Rx R&D Myths*.

2. "A War over Drugs," *Economist*.

3. Bush, "State of the Union"; see also "Who Will Build Our Biodefenses?" *Economist*.

4. Bradsher, "Bayer Halves Price"; Pollack, "Drug Makers Wrestle with World's New Rules."

5. Andrews, "Bayer Is Taken Aback."

6. This is analogous to the concept of "styles" that underpin cultural and scientific arenas; see, for example, Harwood, *Styles of Scientific Thought*; Scheler, *Problems of a Sociology of Knowledge*.

7. Von Beyme, "Power Structure in the Federal Republic of Germany."

8. Office of Technology Assessment, "Product Liability and the Pharmaceutical Industry."

9. Jasanoff, *Fifth Branch*; Galambos, *New American State*; Katzenstein, *Industry and Politics in West Germany*.

10. Pharmaceutical Research and Manufacturers of America, *Pharmaceutical Industry Profile 2003*.

11. Bundesverband der Pharmazeutischen Industrie, *PharmaDaten 2002*; Verband Forschender Arzneimittelhersteller, *Statistics 2002*.

12. Pharmaceutical Research and Manufacturers of America, *Pharmaceutical Industry Profile 2002*.

13. Sullivan, "Pro Pharma."

14. Pharmaceutical Research and Manufacturers of America, *Pharmaceutical Industry Profile 2000*.

15. Dukes, "Regulation of Drugs."

16. DiMasi, "New Drug Innovation."

17. Thayer, "Major Drug Firms Eke Out Increases."

18. Among the best known of the physicians active in the failed 1848 revolution were Rudolph Virchow and Georg Büchner, who later incorporated ethical and political concerns regarding human experimentation into his drama pieces. For more on the 1848 revolution, see Nipperdey, *Germany from Napoleon to Bismarck*, 350–55, 527–98.

19. Burrow, *AMA*, 1–26.

20. Starr, *Social Transformation of American Medicine*.

21. Latour, *Science in Action*, 202.

22. For more on standardization and the construction of "universality" along the spectrum from laboratory testing to real-world application, see Bowker and Star, *Sorting Things Out*; Timmermans and Berg, "Standardization in Action"; Timmermans and Leiter, "Redemption of Thalidomide"; Mallard, "Compare, Standardize and Settle Agreement"; Abraham and Reed, "Progress, Innovation and Regulatory Science."

23. Latour, *Pasteurization of France*, 220; Law and Callon, "Life and Death of an Aircraft."

24. Smith and Wynne, *Expert Evidence*; Latour and Woolgar, *Laboratory Life*.

25. Bijker, Hughes, and Pinch, *Social Construction of Technological Systems*; Collins and Pinch, *Golem*.

26. For more on the interpretive flexibility built into clinical research, see Richards, *Vitamin C and Cancer*; Epstein, *Impure Science*; Marks, *Progress of Experiment*; Marks, "Notes from the Underground."

27. For analogous findings from studies of environmental regulation, see Brickman, Jasanoff, and Ilgen, *Controlling Chemicals*; Vogel, *National Styles of Regulation*.

28. Wiener, "Managing the Iatrogenic Risks of Risk Management."

29. Temin, *Taking Your Medicine*; see also Eisner, *Regulatory Politics in Transition*; Stigler, "Theory of Economic Regulation."

30. Price, *Scientific Estate*.

31. Hart, *Forged Consensus*; Smith, *American Science Policy since World War II*.

32. Jasanoff, "Acceptable Evidence."

33. Jasanoff, *Risk Management and Political Culture*; Graham and Wiener, *Risk versus Risk*.

34. Epstein, *Impure Science*.

35. Starr, *Social Transformation of American Medicine*, 17–29, 420–50.

36. Katzenstein, *Policy and Politics in West Germany*, 15–35; Streeck, "Between Pluralism and Corporatism."

37. Katzenstein, *Industry and Politics in West Germany*, 5–13, 307–16.

38. Katzenstein, "United Germany in an Integrating Europe."

39. Jasanoff, "American Exceptionalism"; Sagar, Daemmrich, and Ashiya, "Tragedy of the Commoners."

Chapter Two

1. Anderson, *Health of a Nation*.

2. Sinclair, *Jungle*.

3. Quoted in Young, *Pure Food*, 192–93.

4. U.S. Congress, "An Act for Preventing," 34 *U.S. Statutes* 768. For more on the 1906 Drug Law see Liebenau, *Medical Science and Medical Industry*.

5. The FDA was moved from the Department of Agriculture to the Federal Security Agency in 1940, then to the Department of Health, Education, and Welfare in 1953, before settling in the Department of Health and Human Services in 1979.

6. Young, *Medical Messiahs*; Swann, "Sure Cure."

7. Cavers, "Food, Drug, and Cosmetic Act of 1938."

8. Lamb, *American Chamber of Horrors*; Kay, "Regulating Beauty."

9. Jackson, *Food and Drug Legislation in the New Deal*.

10. Calvery and Klumpp, "Toxicity for Human Beings."

11. Federal Food, Drug, and Cosmetic Act of 25 June 1938, §505.

12. Marks, *Progress of Experiment*, 73–77.

13. Ibid., 72.

14. Lear, "Taking the Miracle out of the Miracle Drugs"; Speaker, "From 'Happiness Pills' to 'National Nightmare.'"

15. Senate Subcommittee on Antitrust and Monopoly, *Administered Prices*.

16. "Drugs—The Price You Pay," *Newsweek*.

17. Harris, *Real Voice*, 157–69.

18. McFadyen, "Thalidomide in America"; Daemmrich, "Tale of Two Experts"; Kirk, *Der Contergan-Fall*.

19. Mintz, "Heroine of FDA."

20. For more on thalidomide's clinical testing and use, see the case study in Chapter 3.

21. Frances Kelsey, "Summary of FDA's Dealings with the William S. Merrell Company," undated (1962), FDA Files, AF1-542, Accession 72A 2957.

22. Frances Kelsey, "Memorandum of Meeting between Frances Kelsey and Mr. Marshalk," 13 August 1962. FDA Files, AF1-542, Accession 72A 2957.

23. Lear, "Unfinished Story of Thalidomide."

24. Jasanoff, *Fifth Branch*, 153.

25. G. P. Larrick to J. Adriani, 4 June 1963, NLM, Adriani Papers, box 34.

26. Federal Food, Drug, and Cosmetic Act, as amended, §505 (d).

27. *Federal Register* 28 (1963): 179; *Code of Federal Regulations*, Title 21, section 130.3 (1964).

28. Grabowski, *Drug Regulation and Innovation*; Grabowski, Vernon, and Thomas, "Estimating the Effects of Regulation on Innovation"; Peltzman, *Regulation of Pharmaceutical Innovation*.

29. Friedman, "Frustrating Drug Development."

30. Wardell, "'Drug Lag' and American Therapeutics"; Wardell and Lasagna, *Regulation and Drug Development*.

31. Wardell, "Introduction of New Therapeutic Drugs." Practolol was later shown to have serious side effects and was withdrawn from the British and German markets in 1975.

32. Gray, "View from the Capitol."

33. Senate Hearings before the Committee on Labor and Public Welfare, "Regulation of New Drug R&D," 207; Schmidt erred slightly—a congressional hearing was held concerning the non-approval of thalidomide in which the FDA was praised for withholding market access.

34. Hutt, "Investigations and Reports Respecting FDA Regulation of New Drugs (Part I)"; Hutt, "Investigations and Reports Respecting FDA Regulation of New Drugs (Part II)."

35. Asbury, *Orphan Drugs*; Arno, Bonuck, and Davis, "Rare Diseases, Drug Development, and AIDS."

36. Lerner, *Breast Cancer Wars*.

37. Epstein, *Impure Science*, 208–34.

38. Kramer, "FDA's Callous Response to AIDS."

39. Crimp, *AIDS Demographics*, 83.

40. Stone, "How AIDS Has Changed FDA."

41. *Federal Register* 52 (22 May 1987): 19466; Stone, "How AIDS Has Changed FDA."

42. *Federal Register* 53 (21 October 1988): 41516; *Federal Register* 55 (21 May 1990): 20856.

43. *Federal Register* 57 (15 April 1992): 13250; Levi, "Unproven AIDS Therapies."

44. *Federal Register* 57 (11 December 1992): 58942; Epstein, *Impure Science*, 270–76.

45. Kaitin, "Approval Times for New Drugs"; Hileman, "FDA Walks a Fine Line."

46. Hunt, "Prescription Drugs and Intellectual Property."

47. Kaitin, "Prescription Drug User Fee Act of 1992"; Golodner, "U.S. Food and Drug Administration Modernization Act of 1997."

48. Mintzes, "Influence of Direct-to-Consumer Pharmaceutical Advertising"; Rosenthal, "Promotion of Prescription Drugs to Consumers."

49. Datamonitor, *Outlook for Direct-to-Consumer Marketing*, 12.

50. Ridder, *Im Spiegel der Arznei*, 107–21.

51. Murswieck, *Die staatliche Kontrolle der Arzneimittelsicherheit*, 267–79.

52. "Stopverordnung," 11 February 1943, Bundesarchiv Koblenz, B142 (Bundesministerium für Gesundheitswesen), 1432 Arzneimittelgesetzgebung.

53. *Reichsgesetzblatt*. I, 99.

54. Goebbels, "Sportpalastrede" (18 February 1943), cited in Riess, *Joseph Goebbels*, 350–56.

55. Weingart, Kroll, and Bayertz, *Rasse, Blut und Gene*; Proctor, *Racial Hygiene*.

56. Grunwald, "Verbot der Herstellung neuer Arzneifertigwaren," 167.

57. Katzenstein, *Industry and Politics in West Germany*; Stokes, *Divide and Prosper*.

58. Arbeitsgemeinshaft Pharmazeutische Industrie to Ministerialdirektor Prof. Dr. Redeker, 22 May 1950, Bundesarchiv Koblenz, B142 (Bundesministerium für Gesundheitswesen), 1432 Arzneimittelgesetzgebung.

59. Bundesminister des Innern to Präsident des Deutschen Bundestages, 30 January 1951, Bundesarchiv Koblenz, B142 (Bundesministerium für Gesundheitswesen), 1432 Arzneimittelgesetzgebung.

60. Von Blanc, "Herstellung neuer Spezialitäten verboten!"; Riederer and Lauer, "Nochmals die Stopverordnung."

61. "Nichtigkeit der Verordnung über die Herstellung von Arzneifertigwaren vom 11. Februar 1943."

62. "Der Regierungsentwurf des Arzneimittelgesetzes," *Die Pharmazeutische Industrie*. The CDU proposal from 29 January 1959 was based largely on a 1956 bill written by the Interior Ministry. See Bundesminister des Innern, "Referentenentwurf des Gesetzes über den Verkehr mit Arzneimitteln."

63. Stapel, *Die Arzneimittelgesetze 1961 und 1976*, 270–74; Kirk, *Der Contergan-Fall*.

64. Koll, "Fragen der experiementellen Teratologie"; Deutsche Gesellschaft für Innere Medizin, "Richtlinien für die klinische Prüfung von Arzneimitteln."

65. "Zweites Gesetz zur Änderung des Arzneimittelgesetzes vom Bundestag verabschiedet," *Pharmazeutische Zeitung*.

66. Arzneimittelkommission der deutschen Ärzteschaft, "Richtlinien für die Bewertung von Veröffentlichungen"; Sturm, "Mitteilungen des Vorstandes der Deutschen Gesellschaft für innere Medizin."

67. Kathe, "Empfehlungen zum Arzneimittelwesen."

68. 65/65/EWG (26 January 1965); Laar, "Versuche einer Harmonisierung"; Bel, "Die Entwicklung der pharmazeutischen Gesetzgebung."

69. Bundesverband der Pharmazeutischen Industrie, "Referentenentwurf eines Gesetzes zur Neuordnung des Arzneimittelrechts—12.Dezember 1973—Vorläufige Stellungnahme"; Bundesver-

band der Pharmazeutischen Industrie, "Referentenentwurf eines Gesetzes zur Neuordnung des Arzneimittelrechts—12.Dezember 1973"; "Arzneimittel: 3. Arzneimittelgesetzgebung," *Deutsches Ärzteblatt.*

70. "Pharma-Industrie warnt vor Bürokratismus auf dem Arzneimittelmarkt," *Deutsches Ärzteblatt.*

71. "Große Niederlage," *Der Spiegel.*

72. *Arzneimittelgesetz* (Stand: 24 August 1976), §22 (1), (2).

73. Ibid., §24 (1) 3.

74. Fülgraff, "Arzneimittelgesetz."

75. Frankenberg, "Germany: The Uneasy Triumph of Pragmatism."

76. Altman, *Power and Community*, 100–101.

77. Ibid., 74. Altman refers to the book, Salmen, *ACT-UP: Feuer unterm Arsch.*

78. Sander, "Positionspapier des Bundesverbandes der Pharmazeutischen Industrie."

79. Bundesverband der Pharmazeutischen Industrie, *Gesetz über den Verkehr mit Arzneimitteln,* §28.

80. Becker, "Zulassungsstau."

81. Becker, "HIV: Ausschuß oder Kommission?"; Westhoff, "Der Seehofer Skandal."

82. Datamonitor, *Outlook for Direct-to-Consumer Marketing,* 79.

Chapter Three

1. Marks, *Progress of Experiment,* 197–228; Matthews, *Quantification and the Quest for Medical Certainty,* 131–40; Helmchen and Winau, *Versuche mit Menschen.*

2. Latour, "Give Me a Laboratory."

3. Timmermans and Berg, "Standardization in Action."

4. Bull, "Historical Development of Clinical Therapeutic Trials"; Dowling, "Emergence of the Cooperative Clinical Trial"; Shapiro and Shapiro, *Powerful Placebo,* 123–26.

5. Silverman and Chalmers, "Sir Austin Bradford Hill," 102.

6. Yoshioka, "Streptomycin, 1946," 177–80.

7. Winkle, Harwick, Calvery, and Smith, "Laboratory and Clinical Appraisal of New Drugs." For a discussion of the FDA's crusading culture in the 1940s and 1950s, see Marks, *Progress of Experiment.*

8. Martini, *Methodenlehre der therapeutischen Untersuchung*; Martini, *Methodenlehre der therapeutisch-klinischen Forschung.* Subsequent citations refer to the revised 1947 edition.

9. Hill, *Principles of Medical Statistics*; Hill, "Clinical Trial," *British Medical Bulletin*; Hill, "Clinical Trial," *New England Journal of Medicine*; Gold et al., "Xanthines"; Mainland, "Statistics in Clinical Research"; Reid, "Statistics in Clinical Research."

10. Martini, *Methodenlehre,* 3.

11. Ibid., 15.

12. Pross, "Introduction," 2.

13. Jachertz, "Phasen der 'Vergangenheitsbewältigung,' " 275.

14. Marrus, "Nuremberg Doctors' Trial"; Weindling, "Origins of Informed Consent."

15. Diepgen, *Die Heilkunde und der ärztlichen Beruf.*

16. Passages described here are identified in Proctor, *Racial Hygiene,* 304.

17. Martini, "Einseitigkeit und Mitte in der Medizin," 23–28.

18. Marks, "Notes from the Underground."

19. Hobby, *Penicillin: Meeting the Challenge,* 171–97.

20. Mahoney, *Merchants of Life,* 241.

21. Mines, *Pfizer: An Informal History,* 107–21; Mahoney, *Merchants of Life,* 237–52.

22. E. King to Chas. Pfizer & Company, 9 March 1951, FDA Files, AF 12–118.

23. Mahoney, *Merchants of Life*, 243.

24. Bauer et al., "Clinical and Experimental Observations with Terramycin."

25. Blake et al., "Clinical Observations on Terramycin."

26. Ross, "Use of Controls in Medical Research."

27. Blake et al., "Clinical Observations on Terramycin," 498–9.

28. King et al., "Clinical Observations"; see also E. King to Chas. Pfizer & Co., 23 March 1950, FDA Files, AF 12–118; E. King to Chas. Pfizer & Company, 12 July 1950, FDA Files, AF 12–118.

29. H. Welch to G. Hobby (Pfizer), 23 December 1949, FDA Files, AF 12–118.

30. McFadyen, "FDA's Regulation and Control of Antibiotics in the 1950s."

31. Lear, "Certification of Antibiotics."

32. "Terramycin, ein neues Antibiotikum," *Neue Medizinische Welt*.

33. Personal communication from Ruth Linck, Boehringer Ingelheim GmbH, Firmen- und Familienarchiv, 11 March 1997.

34. C. H. Boehringer to Bundesminister des Innern, 23 May 1951, Boehringer.

35. C. H. Boehringer to Professor Dr. Redeker, 19 April 1951, Boehringer.

36. Dr. Nieder to Bundesinnenministerium, 4 June 1951, Bundesarchiv Koblenz, B142 (Bundesministerium für Gesundheitswesen).

37. Doctor R. Burkhardt to the "Scientific Division of the Company Boehringer / Ingelheim," undated (1951), Bundesarchiv Koblenz, B142 (Bundesministerium für Gesundheitswesen).

38. For early case reports, see McBride, "Thalidomide and Congenital Abnormalities"; Lenz, "Kindliche Missbildungen"; Wiedebach, "Totale Phokomelie." For a listing of nearly 1,500 articles and monographs published on thalidomide between 1963 and 1997, see Patrias, Gordner, and Groft, *Thalidomide: Potential Benefits and Risks*.

39. Estimates come from tallies in Bundesarchiv Koblenz, B142—1826 (Bundesverband der Eltern körpergeschädigter Kinder), and U.S. Food and Drug Administration, New Drug Application 12-611: Kevadon (Thalidomide), volume 1; see also Kirk, *Der Contergan-Fall*.

40. "Arzneimittel: Gefahr im Verzuge," *Der Spiegel*.

41. Ibid.; Monser, *Contergan / Thalidomid*, 36.

42. Stephens and Brynner, *Dark Remedy*, 15.

43. Wenzel and Wenzel, *Der Contergan-Prozeß*; Taussig, "A Study of the German Outbreak of Phocomelia."

44. Kirk, *Der Contergan-Fall*, 61. According to Hennig Sjöström, a Swedish lawyer who represented victims, Grünenthal covered up early reports of adverse reactions; see Sjöström and Nilsson, *Thalidomide and the Power of the Drug Companies*, 71–110. Frenkel eventually published an article outlining eleven types of nerve damage that resulted from Contergan use; Frenkel, "Contergan-Nebenwirkungen."

45. This sequence of events is taken from Lenz's testimony in a court case seven years later. See testimony of W. Lenz, *Contergan-Prozeß*, 12 August 1968, 32, IGM.

46. "Mißgeburten durch Tabletten?" *Welt am Sonntag*.

47. Lenz, "Thalidomide and Congenital Abnormalities."

48. "Arzneimittel: Gefahr im Verzuge," 88.

49. Böhm, *Die Entschädigung der Contergan-Kinder*, 14–30; Gemballa, *Der dreifache Skandal*.

50. Rueschemeyer, *Lawyers and Their Society*.

51. Fleming, "Drug Injury Compensation Plans."

52. Testimony of Heinzler, *Contergan-Prozeß*, 11 November 1968, 26 (page 8098 of complete transcript), IGM.

53. Ibid., 40a (page 8116 of complete transcript), IGM.

54. Testimony of Vorlaender, *Contergan-Prozeß*, 19 November 1968, 6 (page 8501 of complete transcript), IGM.

55. Ibid., 13 (page 8506 of complete transcript), IGM.

56. Granitza, "Contergan-Verfahren."

57. Food and Drug Administration, "For Immediate Release," 23 August 1962, FDA Files, AF 1-542, Accession 72A 2957.

58. W. Larkin to Hubert Humphrey, 25 September 1964, New Drug Application 12611: Kevadon (Thalidomide), v. 1.

59. Oldham, Kelsey, and Geiling, *Essentials of Pharmacology*.

60. Kelsey, "Denial of Approval for Thalidomide in the U.S."

61. F. O. Kelsey quoted in McFadyen, "Thalidomide in America," 80.

62. F. Kelsey, "Kevadon (thalidomide)—NDA 12-611: Summary Report," 14 November 1960, New Drug Application 12611: Kevadon (Thalidomide), v. 1.

63. Frances Kelsey, "Summary of FDA's Dealings with the William S. Merrell Company," undated memo, 1961, FDA Files, AF 1-542, Accession 72A 2957.

64. Florence, "Is Thalidomide to Blame?"

65. F. O. Kelsey quoted in Knightley et al., *Suffer the Children*, 79.

66. Beecher, "Ethics and Clinical Research."

67. Beecher, *Measurement of Subjective Responses*, 247.

68. Mintz, "Heroine of FDA Keeps Bad Drug off Market"; "Drug Market Guardian: Frances Oldham Kelsey," *New York Times*.

69. B. Vos to K. Milstead, 30 November 1962, FDA Files, AF 1-542, Accession 72A 2957.

70. Lear, "Unfinished Story of Thalidomide."

71. Food and Drug Administration, "For Immediate Release," 23 August 1962, FDA Files, AF 1-542, Accession 72A 2957.

72. Crout, "R&D Process."

73. Novartis, "Novartis. We're with you . . . for life."

74. Heberden, "Some Account of a Disorder in the Breast."

75. Aronowitz, *Making Sense of Illness*, 85–94.

76. Payer, *Medicine and Culture*, 74–100.

77. Vos, *Drugs Looking for Diseases*, 196–206.

78. Ibid., 157–67.

79. Rhein-Pharma, *Dociton*, 4.

80. Gersmeyer and Spitzbarth, "Beta-Rezeptorenblockade."

81. "Arzneimittel: 3. Prüfung von Arzneimitteln," *Deutsches Ärzteblatt*.

82. Gersmeyer and Spitzbarth, "Beta-Rezeptorenblockade," 779.

83. Bender et al., "Behandlung tachykarder Rhythmusstörungen."

84. Klepzig, "Die konservative Therapie der Angina Pectoris."

85. One such study was carried out using 109 patients in the St. Barnabas Hospital of Staten Island: "Präparate-kombinations günstig bei Angina Pectoris," *Deutsches Ärzteblatt*.

86. Lydtin, "Die Bedeutung der ß-Blocker für die Hochdruckbehandlung."

87. Griffin and Weber, "Voluntary Systems of Adverse Reaction Reporting."

88. C. Steichele, "Sehr verehrte Frau Doktor / Sehr geerhter Herr Doktor," 26 July 1974, AkdÄ.

89. "Studien und Einteilung der in Deutschland beobachteten Fälle von Practolol-Nebenwirkungen," AkdÄ.

90. C. Steichele to K. Kimbel, 5 February 1975, AkdÄ.

91. Arzneimittelkommission der Deutschen Ärzteschaft, "Zweiter Warnhinweis zu Practolol."

92. Gieryn, "Boundaries of Science," 393; see also Gieryn, *Cultural Boundaries of Science: Credibility on the Line*, 12–18; Jasanoff, "Contested Boundaries in Policy-Relevant Science"; Jasanoff, *Fifth Branch*, 76–83, 156–60.

93. J. Jennings to H. Cmojla, 27 October 1969, FDA Files, AF 19-003, Accession 88-78-7.

94. Ibid., 2.

95. A. Kattus to R. Egeberg, 30 December 1969, FDA Files, AF 19-003, Accession 88-80-40.

96. "Memorandum of Conference," 17 April 1970, FDA Files, AF 19-003, Accession 88-80-40.

97. Ibid., 4.

98. E. Belton to H. Perdue, 4 May 1973, FDA Files, AF 19-003, Accession 88-80-40.

99. "FDA Approves Propranolol in Angina Pectoris," *FDA Drug Bulletin*.

100. Ayerst Laboratories, Advertisement.

101. J. Richard Crout to H. Perdue, 22 December 1974, FDA Files, AF 19-003, Accession 88-82-22.

102. Memorandum of meeting between FDA and Ayerst Laboratories, 10 September 1976, FDA Files, AF1 19-003, Accession 88-83-77.

103. Latour, *Science in Action*, 245.

104. Porter, *Trust in Numbers*, 203.

Chapter Four

1. Langbein, Weiss, and Werner, *Gesunde Geschäfte*, 117–48; Neuhaus, "Versuche mit kranken Menschen."

2. Robert Gallo became embroiled in a very public controversy with Luc Montagnier over priority to the discovery of the retrovirus HIV as the root cause of AIDS. For a critical description of Gallo's role in the early years of the AIDS crisis, see Shilts, *And the Band Played On*.

3. Gallo, *Virus Hunting*, 92–94.

4. Löwy, *Between Bench and Bedside*, 124–34.

5. Rosenberg, "Clinical Immunotherapy Studies."

6. Lueck, "Cetus Charting a Broad Course."

7. Rosenberg and Barry, *Transformed Cell*; see also Rabinow, *Making PCR*, 76–78.

8. Bylinsky, "Science Scores a Cancer Breakthrough."

9. Clark et al., "Search for a Cure."

10. Slutsker, "Look before you speak."

11. Lote et al., "High-Dose Recombinant Interleukin-2." The critical review was published in the same issue: Moertel, "On Lymphokines, Cytokines, and Breakthroughs."

12. Moertel, "On Lymphokines, Cytokines, and Breakthroughs," 3141.

13. Lunzer, "Trials of a Cancer Drug," 33.

14. Teitelman, *Gene Dreams*, 186–97.

15. For an example of the sort of clinical trial that advisory committee members criticized for lacking precise definitions of the cancer source and type, see Rosenberg et al., "Experience with the Use of High-Dose Interleukin-2."

16. Culliton, "Cetus's Costly Stumble on IL-2," 21.

17. Keating and Cambrosio, "From Screening to Clinical Research"; Joffe and Weeks, "Views of American Oncologists about the Purposes of Clinical Trials."

18. Food and Drug Administration, "Summary for Basis of Approval: Aldesleukin," 5 May 1992, 14, PLA Reference No. 88-0660.

19. Chiron Corporation, "Proleukin: Package Insert," 1.

20. Food and Drug Administration, "Summary for Basis of Approval: Aldesleukin," 5 May 1992, 2.

21. Hamilton, "Heartbreak and Triumph in Biotech Land," 33.

22. A typical two-phase treatment requires thirty vials of the drug and cost around $11,000 in 1993. The price had risen to $19,000 by 2000. Jenish, "A Risky Treatment."

23. Food and Drug Administration, "Summary for Basis of Approval: Aldesleukin," 5 May 1992, 19-20.

24. Oncologic Drugs Advisory Committee, Meeting # 55, 11.

25. Neeman, "BLA Supplement 97–0501, Proleukin (IL-2) in Metastatic Melanoma," 8.

26. Oncologic Drugs Advisory Committee, Meeting # 55, 97.

27. Ibid., 121–22.

28. Dembner et al., "Public Research, Private Profit."

29. Jasanoff, "Product, Process, or Programme."

30. Bachtler, "Court Blocks German Biotech Plant"; Dolata, *Internationales Innovations-management*, 7–14; Hickel, "Arzneimittel und Gentechnik."

31. Platzer, "Biologische Mediatoren in der Medizin"; Gross, "Interleukine als Mediatoren bei akuten Erkrankungen."

32. "Paul-Martini-Preis für Interleukin-2," *Pharmazeutische Zeitung*.

33. Franks et al., "EuroCetus-Coordinated Clinical Trials."

34. Chiron, *Proleukin: Produktmonographie*.

35. Atzpodien et al., "Home Therapy with Recombinant Interleukin-2"; Atzpodien and Kircher, "Out-patient Use of Recombinant Human Interleukin-2."

36. Steinmetz, "Rekombinantes Interleukin-2"; Ecker-Schlipf, "Immuntherapie des fort-geschrittenen Nierenkarzinoms."

37. Chiron, *Proleukin: Produktmonographie*, 8–12.

38. Ibid., 18.

39. Bundesverband der Pharmazeutischen Industrie, "Chiron: Proleukin."

40. Ibid., 1.

41. "Krebstherapie mit Interleukin-2 noch zu optimieren," *Pharmazeutische Zeitung*.

42. Chiron, "Proleukin: Packungsbeilage für Patienten."

43. Kollek, "Neue Kriterien für die Abschätzung des Risikos"; Gottweis, *Governing Molecules*, 237–61.

44. Chiron, "Proleukin: Produktmonographie," 6–7.

45. Epstein, *Impure Science*, 222–34; Levi, "Unproven AIDS Therapies."

46. Epstein, *Impure Science*, 235–64.

47. Arno and Feiden, *Against the Odds*, 71–73, 207–15; Kolata, "Unorthodox Trials of AIDS Drugs."

48. *Federal Register* 52 (22 May 1987): 19466; *Federal Register* 53 (21 October 1988): 41516; *Federal Register* 55 (21 May 1990): 20856; Stone, "How AIDS Has Changed FDA"; Kessler, "State of the FDA."

49. Merigan, "You Can Teach an Old Dog New Tricks."

50. Andriote, *Victory Deferred*, 197.

51. Food and Drug Administration, "Expanded Access and Expedited Approval."

52. Food and Drug Administration, *From Test Tube to Patient*.

53. National Kidney Cancer Association, *We Have Kidney Cancer*, 51.

54. National Kidney Cancer Association, "13 Steps to World Class Cancer Care."

55. Clinton and Gore, *Reinventing the Regulation of Cancer Drugs*, 3–4.

56. Kramer, *Destiny of Me*, 17.

57. Epstein, *Impure Science*, 293–94.

58. Andriote, *Victory Deferred*, 204.

59. Nowak, "AIDS Researchers, Activists Fight Crisis in Clinical Trials," 1666.

60. Borneman, "AIDS in the Two Berlins."

61. Steinbach, "Bekanntmachung einer Empfehlung über die Mindestanforderungen."

62. Bundesgesundheitsamt, "Nationaler AIDS-Beirat," 1.

63. Rosenbrock, *AIDS: Questions and Lessons for Public Health*, 18.

64. Mbeki, "Speech at the Opening Session of the 13th International AIDS Conference."

65. Cohen, "Protease Inhibitors."

66. Merck, "History of Crixivan—1995."

67. AIDS Project Los Angeles, "Merck announces open-label Crixivan trial," 1.

68. Normal CD4 counts in adults range from 500 to 1,500 cells per cubic milliliter of blood.

69. Naughton, "Drug Lotteries Raise Questions"; Groopman, "Luck of the Draw."

70. Kupec, "FDA Advisory Committee to Discuss Various AIDS Treatments."

71. Antiviral Drugs Advisory Committee, Meeting #22, 24–27.

72. Ibid., 56–58.

73. Ibid., 209.

74. Ibid., 218–19.

75. Ibid., 229.

76. Ibid., 386.

77. Merck, "Livin' It. Tools—Introduction."

78. Merck, "Livin' It. Tools—Personalized Treatment Planner."

79. Antiviral Drugs Advisory Committee, Meeting #22, 368–69.

80. Kupec, "FDA Grants Accelerated Approval to Third Protease Inhibitor."

81. James, "Indinavir (Crixivan) Access and Distribution," 3.

82. "Protease Inhibitors May Increase Blood Glucose in HIV Patients," *FDA Medical Bulletin*.

83. EMEA CPMP, "Crixivan."

84. Ibid. (emphasis added).

85. Will, "Geheimniskrämerie bei der neuen europäischen Zulassungsbehörde," 1.

86. Abraham and Lewis, *Regulating Medicines in Europe*, 80–114.

87. EMEA, *Third General Report 1997*, 21; EMEA, *Fourth General Report 1998*, 19–22.

88. Benzi, "European Medicines Evaluation Agency"; Abraham, "Science and Politics of Medicines Regulation."

89. EMEA, "Decision on rules on access to documents of the EMEA."

90. EMEA, "Interim report on the consultation exercise on transparency and access to documents at the EMEA."

91. "European Medicines Evaluation Agency and the New Licensing Arrangements," *Drug and Therapeutics Bulletin*, 90; see also Brown, "No Place for Secrecy," 3–4.

Chapter Five

1. Latour, "Give Me a Laboratory."

2. Pinch, "Testing," 36 (emphasis in original).

3. Latour, *Pasteurization of France*, 65–67, 162.

4. For more on the AMA Council on Pharmacy and Chemistry, see Marks, *Progress of Experiment*, 32–41.

5. Dowling, "American Medical Association's Policy."

6. Burrow, *AMA*, 108–27; Young, *Medical Messiahs*, 129–57.

7. For a critical review of the AMA's financial dependency on the drug industry, see Starr, *Social Transformation of American Medicine*, 131–34 and 335–79.

8. Maeder, *Adverse Reactions.*

9. Cases were tabulated some years later in "Blood Dyscrasias Associated with Chloramphenicol," *JAMA*; Huguley et al., "Drug-Related Blood Dyscrasias," *JAMA.*

10. Joint Commission on Accreditation of Hospitals, "Reporting of Adverse Drug Reactions."

11. Council on Drugs, "Reporting Adverse Drug Reactions."

12. AMA-BCDSP Pilot Drug Surveillance Study, "Progress Note No. 1," John Adriani Papers, NLM, box 28, folder 2, 1.

13. Ibid.

14. "Suspect and the Innocent," *JAMA.*

15. "FDA Seminar on Adverse Reactions," 6–9 September 1966, John Adriani Papers, NLM, Box 27.

16. Ibid.

17. de Nosaquo, "AMA Registry."

18. U.S. Department of Health, Education, and Welfare, "Doctor: Report Drug Reactions!"

19. AMA-BCDSP Pilot Drug Surveillance Study, "Progress Note No. 1," John Adriani Papers, NLM, box 28, folder 2, 2.

20. Kimbel, "75 Jahre Arzneimittelkommission."

21. "Arzneimittelliste des Deutschen Kongresses für Innere Medizin," *Beilage zum Aerztlichen Vereinsblatt für Deutschland*, 1.

22. Kimbel, "75 Jahre Arzneimittelkommission," 470.

23. Gerst, "Neuaufbau und Konsolidierung."

24. Kimbel, "75 Jahre Arzneimittelkommission," 471.

25. Jacobi et al., "Aufruf zur Sammlung von Erfahrungen," 76.

26. AkdÄ, "Bitte um Mitarbeit aller Ärzte!"

27. "Arzneimittel: 1. Arzneimittelkommission," *Deutsches Ärzteblatt*, 1408.

28. Koller, "Über Möglichkeit und Wirksamkeit."

29. Koll, "Dringende Bitte."

30. "Arzneimittel: 2. Erfassung von Unbekannten Arzneimittelnebenwirkungen," 1525.

31. "Arzneimittel: 3. Prüfung von Arzneimitteln," 1552.

32. Ibid.

33. "Menocil: Wie Zucker," *Der Spiegel*; "Keinen Schuldigen Gefunden," *Die Zeit*, 10.

34. Aschenbrenner, Bock, and Rummel, "Die Arzneimittelkommission," 8.

35. "Arzneimittel: 1. Arzneimittelkommission," 1408.

36. Düppenbecker, "Der 'Rote Hand Brief.'"

37. BÄK, "Verlautbarung des Vorstandes der Bundesärztekammer."

38. Esch, "Food and Drug Administration," 67.

39. Food and Drug Administration, *Adverse Drug Reaction Reporting.*

40. Latour, *Science in Action*, 108–21, 132–44.

41. Latour, *Pandora's Hope*, 311.

42. Esch, "Food and Drug Administration," 69.

43. Forbes et al., "FDA's Adverse Drug Reaction Drug Dictionary."

44. 21 CFR 310.80; *Federal Register* 50 (1985): 7500; see also Sills et al., "Postmarketing Reporting of Adverse Drug Reactions."

45. Abrutyn, "Better Reporting of Adverse Drug Reactions"; Soffer, "Practitioner's Role in Detection"; Rossi and Knapp, "Discovery of New Adverse Drug Reactions."

46. Faich, "Adverse-Drug-Reaction Monitoring," 1589–90.

47. Kessler, "Introducing MEDWatch," 2765.

48. E-Entertainment Survey, "Sex, News and Statistics," 11.

49. FDA, "Medwatch," ⟨https://www.fda.gov/medwatch/report/consumer/consumer.htm⟩.

50. Bates et al., "Incidence of Adverse Drug Events"; Lazarou et al., "Incidence of Adverse Drug Reactions."

51. Moore, *Deadly Medicine*, 281–89.

52. Moore, "FDA Earns Its Own Warning Label"; Willman, "Physician Who Opposes Rezulin Is Threatened by FDA."

53. Wood, Stein, and Woosley, "Making Medicines Safer"; Kleinke and Gottlieb, "Is the FDA Approving Drugs Too Fast?"; Stolberg, "Boom in Medications Brings Rise in Fatal Risks"; Stolberg, "Faulty Warning Labels Add to Risk"; "Bayer droht Millionenklage," *Spiegel Online*.

54. Kohn, Corrigan, and Donaldson, *To Err Is Human*.

55. Task Force on Risk Managment, *Managing the Risks from Medical Product Use*, 69.

56. Hart, "Monitoring Medicines in the Marketplace."

57. Stockhausen, "Erfassen, Sammeln und Auswerten von Arzneimittel-Nebenwirkungen," 2327.

58. Überla, "Perspekitven der Erfassung und Bewertung unerwünschter Arzneimittelwirkungen."

59. Hügel, Fischer, and Kohm, *Pharmazeutische Gesetzeskunde*, 300–304; Höhgrawe, *Implementation der Arzneimittelsicherheitspolitik*, 213–20.

60. Lehr, "Allgemeine Verwaltungsvorschrift," *BAnz*.

61. BPI, *Gesetz über den Verkehr mit Arzneimitteln*, §63 and §63a; Lehr, "Allgemeine Verwaltungsvorschrift," 2570.

62. Deutsch, "Arzneimittelkritik durch Ärztekommissionen."

63. Belz, Olesch, and Schmidt-Voigt, "Die Behandlung des chronischen Vorhofflimmerns."

64. AkdÄ, "Antiarrhythmische Therapie mit Chinidin."

65. A. Thiele to Minden Pharma, 5 August 1993, AkdÄ.

66. J. Beckmann to Minden Pharma, 28 December 1994, AkdÄ.

67. Jörgens et al., "Beschluß im dem verwaltungsgerechtlichen Verfahren der Knoll Deutchland GmbH," 20 January 1995, AkdÄ.

68. Schroiff et al., "Beschluß in dem verwaltungsgerichtlichen Verfahren der Knoll Deutschland GmbH," 20 November 1995, AkdÄ.

69. Cited in Deutsch, "Arzneimittelkritik durch Ärztekommissionen," 389.

70. Burgardt, "Veröffentlichungsbefugnis der Arzneimittelkommission der Deutschen Ärzteschaft," 136.

71. Müller-Oerlinghausen, "Herstellerinteressen oder Patientenschutz?"

72. Dauth, "Risikoinformation hatte Nachspiel im Bundestag."

73. §62 AMG; Art. 1 Nr. 29 Ges. V. 7.6.1998 *BGBL I*, 2649.

Chapter Six

1. Le Carré, *Constant Gardener*, 401.

2. Lewin, "Families Sue Pfizer on Test of Antibiotic."

3. Schmidt, "Monitoring Research Overseas."

4. Keohane, "Governance in a Partially Globalized World"; Putnam, *Bowling Alone*.

5. Foster, "Bundestag im Reichstagsgebäude."

6. Shapin, *Social History of Truth*, 413.

7. Hoff, "Regulatory Environment for the New Millennium," 663.

8. Andersson, "Drug Lag Issue."

9. International Conference on Harmonisation, Steering Committee, "Future of ICH—Revised 2000."

10. Nutley, "Value and Benefits of ICH to Industry."

11. Hoff, "Regulatory Environment."

12. Nightingale, "International Harmonization."

13. International Conference on Harmonisation, "Fourth International Conference on Harmonisation: Background Document."

14. Niklas Luhmann makes this point about social systems more generally; see Luhmann, *Soziale Systeme*.

15. Abraham and Reed, "Progress, Innovation and Regulatory Science."

16. Conradt, *German Polity*, 109.

17. Scott, *Seeing Like a State*, 7–8.

18. Hall, "Personalized Medicine's Bitter Pill"; Arlington et al., *Pharma 2010: The Threshold of Innovation*.

19. DiMasi, "Economics of Pharmaceutical Innovation."

20. Young and Surrusco, *Rx R&D Myths*. See also "Critique of the DiMasi-Tufts Methodology and Other Key Prescription Drug R&D Issues," ⟨http://www.citizen.org/congress/reform/drug—industry/profits/articles.cfm?id=6532⟩, March 2003.

21. Families USA, *Profiting from Pain*.

22. Ezrahi, "Utopian and Pragmatic Rationalism."

23. Dukes, "Seven Pillars of Foolishness," xvii.

Bibliography

Archival Sources and Special Collections

ARZNEIMITTELKOMMISSION DER DEUTSCHEN ÄRZTESCHAFT, RECORDS CENTER, KÖLN, GERMANY

Beckmann, J., to Minden Pharma GmbH, "Abwehr von Arzneimittelrisiken, Stufe II," 28 December 1994.

Jörgens et al. "Beschluß im dem verwaltungsgerechtlichen Verfahren der Knoll Deutchland GmbH gegen die Arzneimittelkommission der Deutschen Ärzteschaft," Verwaltungsgericht Köln, 20 January 1995.

Schroiff et al., "Beschluß in dem verwaltungsgerichtlichen Verfahren der Knoll Deutschland GmbH gegen die Arzneimittelkommission der Deutschen Ärzteschaft," Oberverwaltungsgericht für das Land Nordrhein-Westfalen, 20 November 1995.

Steichele, C. (ICI-Pharma), "Sehr verehrte Frau Doktor / Sehr geerhter Herr Doktor," 26 July 1974.

Steichele, C. (ICI-Pharma), to K. Kimbel (Arzneimittelkommission der Deutschen Ärzteschaft), 5 February 1975.

"Studien und Einteilung der in Deutschland beobachteten Fälle von Practolol-Nebenwirkungen," No author or date available.

Thiele, A., to Minden Pharma GmbH, "Abwehr von Arzneimittelrisiken, Stufe I," 5 August 1993.

BOEHRINGER-INGELHEIM GMBH, CORPORATE ARCHIVES, INGELHEIM, GERMANY

Boehringer, C. H., to Professor Dr. Redeker (Leiter der Abteilung Gesunheitswesen im Bundes-Innenministerium), 19 April 1951.

Boehringer, C. H., to the Bundesminister des Innern, 23 May 1951.

BUNDESARCHIV KOBLENZ

Arbeitsgemeinshaft Pharmazeutische Industrie to Ministerialdirektor Prof. Dr. Redeker, 22 May 1950. Bundesministerium des Innern, B142—Bundesministerium für Gesundheitswesen, 1432: Arzneimittelgesetzgebung, Stop-Verordnung, Rechtsgültigkeit und allgemeine Vorgänge.

Burkhardt, R. (Münchner Universitätsklinik) to "Scientific Division of the Company Boehringer / Ingelheim." B142—Bundesministerium für Gesundheitswesen.

Nieder to the Bundesinnenministerium, 4 June 1951. B142—Bundesministerium für Gesundheitswesen.

Official Answer of the Bundesminister des Innern to the Herrn Präsidenten des Deutschen Bundestages, 30 January 1951. B142—Bundesministerium für Gesundheitswesen, 1432: Arzneimittelgesetzgebung, Stop-Verordnung, Rechtsgültigkeit und allgemeine Vorgänge.

"Stopverordnung vom 11.2.1943," B142—Bundesministerium für Gesundheitswesen, 1432: Arznei-mittelgesetzgebung, Stop-Verordnung, Rechtsgültigkeit und allgemeine Vorgänge.

FOOD AND DRUG ADMINISTRATION, RECORDS CENTER, ROCKVILLE, MD.

Belton, E., to H. Perdue (Ayerst Laboratories), 4 May 1973. FDA Files. AF 19-003. Accession 88-80-40.

Crout, J. Richard, to H. Perdue (Ayerst Laboratories), 22 December 1974. FDA Files. AF 19-003. Accession 88-82-22.

Department of Health, Education, and Welfare, Food and Drug Administration, "For Immediate Release," 23 August 1962, FDA Files. AF 1-542. Accession 72A 2957.

Jennings, J., to H. Cmojla (Ayerst Laboratories), 27 October 1969. FDA Files. AF 19-003. Accession 88-78-7.

Kattus, A. (Division of Cardiology, UCLA), to R. Egeberg (FDA), 30 December 1969. FDA Files AF 19-003. Accession 88-80-40.

Kelsey, F. O. "Kevadon (thalidomide)—NDA 12-611: Summary Report," 14 November 1960. Kevadon (Thalidomide) New Drug Application 12-611, v. 1.

——. "Memorandum of Meeting between Frances Kelsey and Mr. Marshalk, President of Richardson-Merrell," 13 August 1962. FDA Files. AF1-542. Accession 72A 2957.

——. "Summary of FDA's Dealings with the William S. Merrell Company," undated (1962). FDA Files. AF1-542. Accession 72A 2957.

——. "Denial of Approval for Thalidomide in the U.S." Paper presented at the National Library of Medicine, Bethesda, Md., 9 December 1993.

King, E., to Chas. Pfizer & Co. "Approving Terramycin," 23 March 1950. FDA Files. AF 12-118.

——. "Approving Terrabon (Terramycin Elixir)," 12 July 1950. FDA Files. AF 12-118.

——. "Concerns pertaining to the safety of Terramycin," 9 March 1951. FDA Files. AF 12-118.

Larkin, W., to Hubert Humphrey (U.S. Senate), 25 September 1964. New Drug Application 12611: Kevadon (Thalidomide), v. 1.

Memorandum of Conference: Propranolol, 17 April 1970. FDA Files. AF 19-003. Accession 88-80-40.

Memorandum of Meeting between FDA and Ayerst Laboratories, 10 September 1976. FDA Files. AF1 19-003. Accession 88-83-77.

Neeman, T. "BLA Supplement 97-0501, Proleukin (IL-2) in Metastatic Melanoma, Chiron Corporation." FDA Memorandum, 4 November 1997. ⟨http://www.fda.gov⟩. February 2002.

U.S. Department of Health, Education, and Welfare. Food and Drug Administration. "For Immediate Release," 23 August 1962. FDA Files. AF 1-542. Accession 72A 2957.

Vos, B., to K. Milstead (FDA Bureau of Enforcement). "Falsification and Omissions in Wm. S. Merrell's NDA 12-611, Kevadon," 30 November 1962. FDA Files. AF 1-542. Accession 72A 2957.

Welch, H., to G. Hobby (Chas. Pfizer and Co.). "Detailing treatment of patients with Combiotic," 23 December 1949. FDA Files. AF 12-118.

INSTITUT FÜR GESCHICHTE DER MEDIZIN DER FREIEN UNIVERSITÄT BERLIN, BERLIN, GERMANY
Contergan-Prozeß.

NATIONAL LIBRARY OF MEDICINE, BETHESDA, MD., JOHN ADRIANI PAPERS

AMA-BCDSP Pilot Drug Surveillance Study. "Progress Note No. 1," 22 February 1971. Box 28. Folder 2.

Larrick, G. P., to J. Adriani, 4 June 1963. Box 34.

Report to Committee on Adverse Drug Reactions. "FDA Seminars on Adverse Reactions," 6–9 September 1966. Box 27.

Published and Other Materials

Abraham, J. "The Science and Politics of Medicines Regulation." In *The Sociology of Medical Science and Technology*, ed. M. A. Elston, 153–82. Oxford: Blackwell, 1997.

Abraham, J., and G. Lewis. *Regulating Medicines in Europe: Competition, Expertise and Public Health.* London: Routledge, 2000.

Abraham, J., and T. Reed. "Progress, Innovation and Regulatory Science in Drug Development: The Politics of International Standard-Setting." *Social Studies of Science* 32 (2002): 337–69.

Abrutyn, E. "Better Reporting of Adverse Drug Reactions." *Annals of Internal Medicine* 102 (1985): 264–65.

AIDS Project Los Angeles. "Merck Announces Open-Label Crixivan Trial." *Positive Living Newsletter*, August 1995, 1.

AkdÄ. "Bitte um Mitarbeit aller Ärzte!" *Deutsches Ärzteblatt*, 13 July 1963. Reprinted in *Arzneimittelgesetzgebung, Arzneimittelprüfung, Arzneimittelbeobachtung in der Bundesrepublik Deutschland*, ed. Bundesärztekammer, 80–81. Köln: Deutsche Ärzte-Verlag, 1970.

Altman, D. *Power and Community: Organizational and Cultural Responses to AIDS.* London: Taylor & Francis, 1994.

Anderson, O. E. *The Health of a Nation: Harvey W. Wiley and the Fight for Pure Food.* Chicago: University of Chicago Press, 1958.

Andersson, F. "The Drug Lag Issue: The Debate Seen from an International Perspective." *International Journal of Health Services* 22 (1992): 53–72.

Andrews, E. "Bayer Is Taken Aback by the Frenzy to Get Its Drug." *New York Times*, 26 October 2001, A1.

Andriote, J. *Victory Deferred: How AIDS Changed Gay Life in America.* Chicago: University of Chicago Press, 1999.

Antiviral Drugs Advisory Committee, Meeting #22, Holiday Inn, Gaithersburg, Md. (1 March 1996).

Arlington, S., et al. *Pharma 2010: The Threshold of Innovation.* Portsmouth, Hampshire, U.K.: IBM Business Consulting Services, 2003.

Arno, P., and K. Feiden. *Against the Odds: The Story of AIDS Drug Development, Politics and Profits.* New York: HarperCollins Publishers, 1992.

Arno, P., K. Bonuck, and M. Davis. "Rare Diseases, Drug Development, and AIDS: The Impact of the Orphan Drug Act." *Milbank Quarterly* 73 (1995): 231–52.

Aronowitz, R. *Making Sense of Illness: Science, Society, and Disease.* Cambridge: Cambridge University Press, 1988.

"Arzneimittel: Gefahr im Verzuge." *Der Spiegel*, 5 December 1962, 72–90.

"Arzneimittel: 1. Arzneimittelkommission der Deutschen Ärzteschaft." *Deutsches Ärzteblatt* (19 June 1965): 1406–08.

"Arzneimittel: 2. Erfassung von Unbekannten Arzneimittelnebenwirkungen." *Deutsches Ärzteblatt* (15 July 1967): 1524–1526.

"Arzneimittel: 3. Prüfung von Arzneimitteln." *Deutsches Ärzteblatt* (21 May 1969): 1551–1553.

"Arzneimittel: 4. Arzneimittelgesetzgebung." *Deutsches Ärzteblatt* (3 June 1970): 1832.

Arzneimittelgesetz (Stand: 24 August 1976).

Arzneimittelkommission der deutschen Ärzteschaft. "Richtlinien für die Bewertung von Veröffentlichungen, Gutachten und anderen Unterlagen über den therapeutischen Wert von Arzneimitteln." In *Arzneimittelgesetzgebung, Arzneimittelprüfung, Arzneimittel-beobachtung in der Bundesrepublik Deutschland, 1961–1969*, ed. Bundesärztekammer, 63–65. Köln: Deutsches Ärzte-Verlag, 1970.

——. "Zweiter Warnhinweis zu Practolol." *Deutsches Ärzteblatt* 13 (27 March 1975): 859.

——. "Antiarrhythmische Therapie mit Chinidin / Verapamil." *Deutsches Ärzteblatt* 88 (4 July 1991): 2409.

"Arzneimittelliste des Deutschen Kongresses für Innere Medizin." *Beilage zum Aerztlichen Vereinsblatt für Deutschland* 41 (14 May 1912): 1.

Asbury, C. *Orphan Drugs: Medical versus Market Value.* Lexington, Mass.: Lexington Books, 1985.

Aschenbrenner, R., K. D. Bock, and W. Rummel. "Die Arzneimittelkommission als 'Feindattrappe.'" *Deutsches Ärzteblatt* 68 (2 January 1971): 7–9.

Atzpodien, J., and H. Kircher. "The Out-Patient Use of Recombinant Human Interleukin-2 and Interferon Alpha-2b in Advanced Malignancies." *European Journal of Cancer* 27 (1991): S88–S92.

Atzpodien, J., et al. "Home Therapy with Recombinant Interleukin-2 and Interferon Alpha-2b in Advanced Human Malignancies." *Lancet* 335 (1990): 1509–12.

Ayerst Laboratories. Advertisement. *JAMA* (4 November 1974): 675–79.

Bachtler, B. "Court Blocks German Biotech Plant." *Science* 246 (1989): 881.

Bates, D., et al. "Incidence of Adverse Drug Events." *JAMA* 274 (1995): 29–34.

Bauer, R., et al. "Clinical and Experimental Observations with Terramycin in Certain Rickettsial and Bacterial Infections." *Annals of the New York Academy of Sciences* 53 (1950): 395–406.

"Bayer droht Millionenklage." *Spiegel Online*, 8 August 2001. ⟨http://www.spiegel.de/wirtschaft/0,1518,149165,00.html⟩. August 2001.

Becker, J. "Zulassungsstau: Kein Ende in Sicht." *Pharmazeutische Zeitung* 137 (20 February 1992): 17–18.

——. "HIV: Ausschuß oder Kommission?" *Pharmazeutische Zeitung* 138 (28 October 1993): 3444.

Beecher, H. *Measurement of Subjective Responses: Quantitative Effects of Drugs.* New York: Oxford University Press, 1959.

——. "Ethics and Clinical Research." *New England Journal of Medicine* 274 (1966): 1354–60.

Bel, N. "Die Entwicklung der pharmazeutischen Gesetzgebung in der EWG." *Pharmazeutische Industrie* 42 (1980): 894–99.

Belz, G., K. Olesch, and J. Schmidt-Voigt. "Die Behandlung des chronischen Vorhofflimmerns mit einer Kombination von Chinidin und Verapamil." *Medizinische Welt* 21 (1970): 1670–72.

Bender, F., et al. "Behandlung tachykarder Rhythmusstörungen des Herzens durch Beta-Rezeptorenblockade des Atrioventrikulargewebes." *Die Medizinische Welt* 17 (1966): 1120–23.

Benzi, G. "The European Medicines Evaluation Agency: Role of Experts in Drug Assessment." *Trends in Pharmacological Sciences* 16 (1995): 409–12.

Bijker, W. E., T. P. Hughes, and T. J. Pinch, eds. *The Social Construction of Technological Systems.* Cambridge: MIT Press, 1989.

Blake, F., et al. "Clinical Observations on Terramycin." *Yale Journal of Biology and Medicine* 22 (1950): 495–507.

"Blood Dyscrasias Associated with Chloramphenicol (Chloromycetin) Therapy." *JAMA* 172 (30 April 1960): 2044–45.

Böhm, D. *Die Entschädigung der Contergan-Kinder.* Bonn: Vorländer Verlag, 1973.

Borneman, J. "AIDS in the Two Berlins." In *AIDS: Cultural Analysis, Cultural Activism*, ed. D. Crimp. Cambridge: MIT Press, 1988.

Bowker, G., and S. L. Star. *Sorting Things Out: Classification and Its Consequences.* Cambridge: MIT Press, 1999.

Bradsher, K. "Bayer Halves Price for Cipro, but Rivals Offer Drugs Free." *New York Times*, 26 October 2001, B1.

Brickman, R., S. Jasanoff, and T. Ilgen. *Controlling Chemicals: The Politics of Regulation in Europe and the United States.* Ithaca: Cornell University Press, 1985.

Brown, P. "No Place for Secrecy." *Scrip Magazine*, December 1993, 3–4.

Bull, J. "The Historical Development of Clinical Therapeutic Trials." *Journal of Chronic Diseases* 10 (1959): 218–48.

Bundesärztekammer. "Verlautbarung des Vorstandes der Bundesärztekammer." *Deutsches Ärzteblatt* (13 July 1968): 1570.

Bundesgesundheitsamt. "Nationaler AIDS-Beirat lehnt Heimtests zur HIV-Diagnostik ab." *Pressemitteilung* 58 (9 July 1996): 1.

Bundesminister des Innern. "Referentenentwurf des Gesetzes über den Verkehr mit Arzneimitteln (Arzneimittelgesetz)." *Die Pharmazeutische Industrie* 18 (1956): 174–85.

Bundesverband der Pharmazeutischen Industrie. "Referentenentwurf eines Gesetzes zur Neuordnung des Arzneimittelrechts—12.Dezember 1973—Vorläufige Stellungnahme des Bundesverbandes der Pharmazeutischen Industrie." *Die Pharmazeutische Industrie* 36 (1974): 161–78.

———. "Referentenentwurf eines Gesetzes zur Neuordnung des Arzneimittelrechts—12. Dezember 1973." *Die Pharmazeutische Industrie* 36 (1974): 313–16.

———. "Chiron: Proleukin." *Fachinformation.* Aulendorf: BPI, 1994.

———. *Gesetz über den Verkehr mit Arzneimitteln (AMG).* Aulendorf: Editio Cantor Verlag, 1997.

———. *PharmaDaten 2000.* Frankfurt am Main: BPI, 2000.

———. *PharmaDaten 2002.* Berlin: BPI, 2002.

Burgardt, C. "Veröffentlichungsbefugnis der Arzneimittelkommission der Deutschen Ärzteschaft." *Pharma Recht* (May 1996): 136–41.

Burrow, J. *AMA: Voice of American Medicine.* Baltimore: Johns Hopkins University Press, 1963.

Bush, G. State of the Union Address. *New York Times,* 30 January 2003.

Bylinsky, G. "Science Scores a Cancer Breakthrough." *Fortune,* 25 November 1985, 16–21.

Calvery, H. O., and T. G. Klumpp. "The Toxicity for Human Beings of Diethylene Glycol with Sulfanilamide." *Southern Medical Journal* 32 (1939): 1106–07.

Cavers, D. F. "The Food, Drug, and Cosmetic Act of 1938: Its Legislative History and Its Substantive Provisions." *Law and Contemporary Problems* 6 (1939): 2–42.

Chiron. "Proleukin: Package Insert." May 1992.

———. "Proleukin: Packungsbeilage für Patienten." December 1994.

———. *Proleukin: Produktmonographie.* Amsterdam: Chiron Corporation, 1995.

Clark, M., et al. "Search for a Cure." *Newsweek,* 16 December 1985, 60–65.

Clinton, B., and A. Gore. *Reinventing the Regulation of Cancer Drugs: Accelerating Approval and Expanding Access.* Washington, D.C.: Government Printing Office, 1996.

Cohen, J. "Protease Inhibitors: A Tale of Two Companies." *Science* 272 (28 June 1996): 1882–83.

Collins, H. M., and T. J. Pinch. *The Golem.* Cambridge: Cambridge University Press, 1993.

Conradt, D. *The German Polity.* New York: Longman, 1993.

Council on Drugs. "Reporting Adverse Drug Reactions." *JAMA* 196 (2 May 1966): 143–44.

Crimp, D. *AIDS Demographics.* Seattle: Bay Press, 1990.

Crout, J. R. "R&D Process: Decision Making." In *Drugs and Health: Economic Issues and Policy Objectives,* ed. R. Helms. Washington, D.C.: American Enterprise Institute, 1981.

Culliton, B. "Cetus's Costly Stumble on IL-2." *Science* 250 (1990): 20–21.

Daemmrich, A. "A Tale of Two Experts: Thalidomide and Political Engagement in the United States and West Germany." *Social History of Medicine* 15 (2002): 137–58.

Datamonitor. *The Outlook for Direct-to-Consumer Marketing: Maximizing the Return on Your Investment.* London: Reuters Business Insight, 2002.

Dauth, S. "Risikoinformation hatte Nachspiel im Bundestag." *Deutsches Ärzteblatt* 93 (26 July 1996): 1939.

Dembner, A., et al. "Public Research, Private Profit: Public Handouts Enrich Drug Makers, Scientists." *Boston Globe,* 5 April 1998, A1, A32–33.

de Nosaquo, N. "AMA Registry on Adverse Reactions." *Journal of Chemical Documentation* 9 (May 1969): 59–65.

Deutsch, E. "Arzneimittelkritik durch Ärztekommissionen." *Versicherungsrecht* 48 (1997): 389–432.

Deutsche Gesellschaft für Innere Medizin. "Richtlinien für die klinische Prüfung von Arzneimitteln." In *Arzneimittelgesetzgebung, Arzneimittelprüfung, Arzneimittel-beobachtung in der Bundesrepublik Deutschland, 1961–1969*, ed. Bundesärztekammer, 53–61. Köln: Deutsches Ärzte-Verlag, 1970.

Diepgen, P. *Die Heilkunde und der ärztlichen Beruf.* Munich: J. F. Lehmann, 1938. 2nd ed., Berlin, Urban & Schwarzenberg, 1947.

DiMasi, J. "New Drug Innovation and Pharmaceutical Industry Structure: Trends in the Output of Pharmaceutical Firms." *Drug Information Journal* 34 (2000): 1169–94.

——. "Economics of Pharmaceutical Innovation: New Estimates of New Drug Development Costs." Talk presented at the Tufts Center for the Study of Drug Discovery Policy Forum, 30 November 2001.

Dolata, U. *Internationales Innovationsmanagement: Die deutsche Pharmaindustrie und die Gentechnik.* Hamburg: Hamburger Institut für Sozialforschung, 1994.

Dowling, H. F. "The American Medical Association's Policy on Drugs in Recent Decades." In *Safeguarding the Public: Historical Aspects of Medicinal Drug Control*, ed. J. B. Blake, 123–31. Baltimore: Johns Hopkins University Press, 1970.

——. "The Emergence of the Cooperative Clinical Trial." *Transactions and Studies of the College of Physicians of Philadelphia* 43 (1975): 20–29.

"Drug Market Guardian: Frances Oldham Kelsey." *New York Times*, 2 August 1962, A1.

"Drugs—The Price You Pay." *Newsweek*, 7 December 1959, 87–89.

Dukes, M. N. G. "The Seven Pillars of Foolishness." *Side Effects of Drugs Annual* 8 (1984): xvii–xxiii.

——. "The Regulation of Drugs: Worlds of Difference." *International Journal of Technology Assessment in Health Care* 2 (1986): 629–36.

Düppenbecker, H. "Der 'Rote Hand Brief.'" *Deutsches Ärzteblatt* 89 (30 October 1992): 3642–44.

Ecker-Schlipf, B. "Immuntherapie des fortgeschrittenen Nierenkarzinoms." *Deutsche Apotheker Zeitung* 131 (1991): 1999.

E-Entertainment Survey. "Sex, News and Statistics." *The Economist*, 7 October 2000, 11.

Eisner, M. *Regulatory Politics in Transition.* Baltimore: Johns Hopkins University Press, 1993.

Epstein, S. *Impure Science: AIDS, Activism, and the Politics of Knowledge.* Berkeley: University of California Press, 1996.

Esch, A. "Food and Drug Administration Drug Experience Reporting System." *Journal of Chemical Documentation* 9 (May 1969): 66–70.

European Agency for the Evaluation of Medicinal Products (EMEA). "Decision on rules on access to documents of the EMEA." Luxembourg: European Commission, 1997. ⟨http://www.eudra.org/emea.html⟩. February 2002.

——. "Interim report on the conultation exercise on transparency and access to documents at the EMEA." Luxembourg: European Commission, 1997. ⟨http://www.eudra.org/emea.html⟩. February 2002.

——. Commission on Proprietary Medicinal Products (CPMP). "Crixivan." *European Public Assessment Report.* London: EMEA, October 1997.

——. *Third General Report 1997.* Luxembourg: European Commission, 1998.

——. *Fourth General Report 1998.* Luxembourg: European Commission, 1999.

"European Medicines Evaluation Agency and the New Licensing Arrangements." *Drug and Therapeutics Bulletin* 32 (15 December 1994): 89–90.

Ezrahi, Y. "Utopian and Pragmatic Rationalism: The Political Context of Scientific Advice." *Minerva* 18 (1980): 111–31.

Faich, G. "Adverse-Drug-Reaction Monitoring." *New England Journal of Medicine* 314 (12 June 1986): 1589–92.

Families USA. *Profiting from Pain: Where Prescription Dollars Go.* Washington, D.C.: Families USA, 2002.

"FDA Approves Propranolol in Angina Pectoris." *FDA Drug Bulletin*, January 1974, 1.

Fleming, J. G. "Drug Injury Compensation Plans." *American Journal of Comparative Law* 30 (1982): 297–323.

Florence, A. "Is Thalidomide to Blame?" *British Medical Journal* (31 December 1960): 1954.

Food and Drug Administration. *Adverse Drug Reaction Reporting.* Washington, D.C.: FDA, 1969.

——. "Summary for Basis of Approval: Aldesleukin." PLA Reference No. 88-0660 (5 May 1992).

——. *From Test Tube to Patient: New Drug Development in the United States.* Washington, D.C.: Government Printing Office, 1995.

——. Office of Special Health Issues. "Expanded Access and Expedited Approval of New Therapies Related to HIV / AIDS." ⟨http: / / www.fda.gov⟩. February 2002.

Forbes, M., et al. "FDA's Adverse Drug Reaction Drug Dictionary and Its Role in Post-Marketing Surveillance." *Drug Information Journal* 20 (1986): 135–45.

Foster, N. "Bundestag im Reichstagsgebäude." In *Die Bauten des Bundes in Berlin, 1991–2000*, ed. Bundesministerium für Verkehr, Bau- und Wohnungswesen, 52–69. Hamburg: Junius Verlag, 2000.

Frankenberg, G. "Germany: The Uneasy Triumph of Pragmatism." In *AIDS in the Industrialized Democracies*, ed. D. Kirp and R. Bayer, 99–133. New Brunswick: Rutgers University Press, 1992.

Franks, C., et al. "EuroCetus-Coordinated Clinical Trials." In *Therapeutic Applications of Interleukin-2*, ed. M. Atkins and J. Mier, 311–25. New York: Marcel Dekker, 1993.

Frenkel, H. "Contergan-Nebenwirkungen." *Deutsche Medizinische Wochenschrift* 86 (6 May 1961): 970–75.

Friedman, M. "Frustrating Drug Development." *Newsweek*, 8 January 1973.

Fülgraff, G. "Arzneimittelgesetz—Anspruch und Wirklichkeit." *Die Pharmazeutische Industrie* 42 (1980): 581–87.

Galambos L., ed. *The New American State: Bureaucracies and Policies since World War II.* Baltimore: Johns Hopkins University Press, 1987.

Gallo, R. *Virus Hunting: AIDS, Cancer, and the Human Retrovirus.* New York: Basic Books, 1991.

Gemballa, G. *Der dreifache Skandal. 30 Jahre nach Contergan: Eine Dokumentation.* Hamburg: Luchterhand Verlag, 1993.

Gersmeyer E., and H. Spitzbarth. "Beta-Rezeptorenblockade in klinischer Pharmakologie und Therapie." *Die Medizinische Welt* 18 (1967): 764–79.

Gerst, T. "Neuaufbau und Konsolidierung: Ärztliche Selbstverwaltung und Interessenvertretung in den drei Westzonen und der Bundesrepublik Deutschland, 1945–1995." In *Geschichte der deutschen Ärzteschaft*, ed. R. Jütte, 195–242. Köln: Deutsche Ärzte-Verlag, 1997.

Gieryn, T. "Boundaries of Science." In *Handbook of Science and Technology Studies*, ed. S. Jasanoff, 393–443. Thousand Oaks, Calif.: Sage Publications, 1995.

——. *Cultural Boundaries of Science: Credibility on the Line.* Chicago: University of Chicago Press, 1999.

Gold, H., et al. "The Xanthines (Theobromine and Aminophylline) in the Treatment of Cardiac Pain." *JAMA* 108 (1937): 2173–79.

Golodner, L. "The U.S. Food and Drug Administration Modernization Act of 1997: Impact on Consumers." *Clinical Therapeutics* 20 Suppl C (1998): C20–25.

Gottweis, H. *Governing Molecules: The Discursive Politics of Genetic Engineering in Europe and the United States.* Cambridge: MIT Press, 1998.

Grabowski, H. *Drug Regulation and Innovation: Empirical Evidence and Policy Options.* Washington, D.C.: American Enterprise Institute, 1976.

Grabowski, H., J. Vernon, and L. Thomas. "Estimating the Effects of Regulation on Innovation: An International Comparative Analysis of the Pharmaceutical Industry." *Journal of Law and Economics* 21 (1978): 133–63.

Graham, J. D., and J. B. Wiener. *Risk versus Risk: Tradeoffs in Protecting Health and the Environment.* Cambridge: Harvard University Press, 1995.

Granitza, A. "Contergan-Verfahren: Konsequenzen für die pharmazeutische Industrie." *Pharmazeutische Industrie* 34 (1972): 409–11.

Gray, W. "The View from the Capitol." In *The Economics of Drug Innovation*, ed. J. Cooper, 17–22. Washington, D.C.: American University, Center for the Study of Private Enterprise, School of Business Administration, 1969.

Griffin, J. P., and J. C. P. Weber. "Voluntary Systems of Adverse Reaction Reporting." In *Medicines: Regulation, Research and Risk*, ed. J. P. Griffin, 217–60. Queens University of Belfast, 1989.

Groopman, J. "Luck of the Draw." *Boston Globe Magazine*, 19 March 2000, 14–24.

Gross, R. "Interleukine als Mediatoren bei akuten Erkrankungen." *Deutsches Ärzteblatt* 82 (1985): 3780–81.

"Große Niederlage." *Der Spiegel*, 17 May 1976, 46–49.

Grunwald, J. "Verbot der Herstellung neuer Arzneifertigwaren." *Die Pharmazeutische Industrie* 6 (1943): 166–69.

Hall, S. "Personalized Medicine's Bitter Pill." *Technology Review* (February 2003): 63–70.

Hamilton, J. "Heartbreak and Triumph in Biotech Land." *Business Week*, 3 February 1992, 33.

Harris, R. *The Real Voice.* New York: Macmillan, 1964.

Hart, C. "Monitoring Medicines in the Marketplace." *Modern Drug Discovery* (June 2000): 40–44.

Hart, D. *Forged Consensus: Science, Technology and Economic Policy in the United States.* Princeton: Princeton University Press, 1998.

Harwood, J. *Styles of Scientific Thought: The German Genetics Community, 1900–1933.* Chicago: University of Chicago Press, 1993.

Heberden, W. "Some Account of a Disorder in the Breast." *Medical Transactions of the College of Physicians of London* 2 (1772): 59–67.

Helmchen, H., and R. Winau, eds. *Versuche mit Menschen.* Berlin: Walter de Gruyter, 1986.

Hickel, E. "Arzneimittel und Gentechnik." *Deutsche Apotheker Zeitung* 128 (1988): 297–303.

Hileman, B. "FDA Walks a Fine Line." *Chemical and Engineering News*, 2 December 2002, 58–65.

Hill, A. B. *Principles of Medical Statistics.* 5th ed. London: Lancet Press, 1950.

——. "The Clinical Trial." *British Medical Bulletin* 7 (1951): 278–82.

——. "The Clinical Trial." *New England Journal of Medicine* 247 (1952): 113–19.

Hobby, G. *Penicillin: Meeting the Challenge.* New Haven: Yale University Press, 1985.

Hoff, S. "The Regulatory Environment for the New Millennium." *Drug Information Journal* 34 (2000): 659–72.

Höhgrawe, U. *Implementation der Arzneimittelsicherheitspolitik durch das Bundesgesundheitsamt.* Baden-Baden: Nomos Verlag, 1992.

Hügel, H., J. Fischer, and B. Kohm. *Pharmazeutische Gesetzeskunde: Textesammlung für Studium und Praxis.* Stuttgart: Deutscher Apotheker Verlag, 1995.

Huguley, C. M., et al. "Drug-Related Blood Dyscrasias." *JAMA* 177 (8 July 1961): 23–26.

Hunt, M. "Prescription Drugs and Intellectual Property Protection." *National Institute for Health Care Management Issue Brief*, August 2002.

Hutt, P. B. "Investigations and Reports Respecting FDA Regulation of New Drugs (Part I)." *Clinical Pharmacology and Therapeutics* 33 (1983): 537–48.

———. "Investigations and Reports Respecting FDA Regulation of New Drugs (Part II)." *Clinical Pharmacology and Therapeutics* 33 (1983): 674–87.

International Conference on Harmonisation. "Fourth International Conference on Harmonisation: Background Document." 16–18 July 1997.

———. Steering Committee. "The Future of ICH—Revised 2000." Statement on the occasion of the Fifth International Conference on Harmonisation, 9 November 2000. ⟨http://www.ifpma .org/ich1.html⟩. April 2003.

Jachertz, N. "Phasen der 'Vergangenheitsbewältigung' in der deutschen Ärzteschaft nach dem Zweiten Weltkrieg." In *Geschichte der detuschen Ärzteschaft*, ed. R. Jütte, 275–88. Köln: Deutsche Ärzte-Verlag, 1997.

Jackson, C. O. *Food and Drug Legislation in the New Deal*. Princeton: Princeton University Press, 1970.

Jacobi, J., et al. "Aufruf zur Sammlung von Erfahrungen über Arzneimittel-Nebenwirkungen." *Deutsches Ärzteblatt*, 5 August 1961. Reprinted in *Arzneimittelgesetzgebung, Arzneimittelprüfung, Arzneimittelbeobachtung in der Bundesrepublik Deutschland*, ed. Bundesärztekammer, 76. Köln: Deutsche Ärzte-Verlag, 1970.

James, J. "Indinavir (Crixivan) Access and Distribution." *AIDS Treatment News*, 5 April 1996.

Jasanoff, S. *Risk Management and Political Culture*. New York: Russell Sage Foundation, 1986.

———. "Contested Boundaries in Policy-Relevant Science." *Social Studies of Science* 17 (1987): 195–230.

———. *The Fifth Branch: Science Advisers as Policymakers*. Cambridge: Harvard University Press, 1990.

———. "American Exceptionalism and the Political Acknowledgement of Risk." *Daedalus* 119 (1990): 61–81.

———. "Acceptable Evidence in a Pluralistic Society." In *Acceptable Evidence: Science and Values in Risk Management*, ed. D. Mayo and R. Hollander, 29–47. New York: Oxford University Press, 1991.

———. "Product, Process, or Programme: Three Cultures and the Regulation of Biotechnology." In *Resistance to New Technology*, ed. M. Bauer, 311–31. Cambridge: Cambridge University Press, 1995.

Jenish, D. "A Risky Treatment." *Maclean's* 106 (22 February 1993): 52–53.

Joffe, S., and J. Weeks. "Views of American Oncologists about the Purposes of Clinical Trials." *Journal of the National Cancer Institute* 94 (2002): 1847–53.

Joint Commission on Accreditation of Hospitals. "Reporting of Adverse Drug Reactions." *Bulletin of the Joint Commission* 39 (August 1965).

Kaitin, K. "The Prescription Drug User Fee Act of 1992 and the New Drug Development Process." *American Journal of Therapeutics* 4 (1997): 167–72.

———. "Approval Times for New Drugs Fell by More than a Year during PDUFA." *Tufts Center for the Study of Drug Development Impact Report* 4 (November/December 2002).

Kathe, H. "Empfehlungen zum Arzneimittelwesen anläßlich der Gesundheitspolitischen Konferenz der SPD." *Die Pharmazeutische Industrie* 33 (1971): 205–18.

Katzenstein, P. *Policy and Politics in West Germany: The Growth of a Semisovereign State*. Philadelphia: Temple University Press, 1987.

———. *Industry and Politics in West Germany: Toward the Third Republic*. Ithaca: Cornell University Press, 1989.

———. "United Germany in an Integrating Europe." In *Tamed Power: Germany in Europe*, ed. P. Katzenstein, 1–48. Ithaca: Cornell University Press, 1997.

Kay, G. "Regulating Beauty: Cosmetics in American Culture from the 1906 Pure Food and Drugs Act to the 1938 Food, Drug, and Cosmetic Act." Ph.D. diss., Yale University, 1997.

Keating, P., and A. Cambrosio. "From Screening to Clinical Research: The Cure of Leukemia and the Early Development of the Cooperative Oncology Groups, 1955–1966." *Bulletin of the History of Medicine* 76 (2002): 299–334.

"Keinen Schuldigen Gefunden: Die Staatsanwaltschaft stellte die Ermittlung gegen die Arzneimittelfirma Cilag ein." *Die Zeit*, 13 November 1970, 10.

Keohane, R. "Governance in a Partially Globalized World." *American Political Science Review* 95 (March 2001): 1–13.

Kessler, D. "Introducing MEDWatch." *JAMA* 269 (1993): 2765–68.

———. "State of the FDA." Text of Remarks Made at the Food and Drug Law Institute, 12 December 1995.

Kimbel, K. "75 Jahre Arzneimittelkommission." *Schleswig-Holsteinisches Ärzteblatt* 8 (1986): 466–71.

King, E., et al. "Clinical Observations on the Use of Terramycin Hydrochloride." *JAMA* 143 (1950): 1–5.

Kirk, B. *Der Contergan-Fall: eine unvermeidbare Arzneimittelkatastrophe?* Stuttgart: Deutsche Apotheker Verlag, 1999.

Kleinke, J., and S. Gottlieb. "Is the FDA Approving Drugs Too Fast?" *British Medical Journal* 317 (1998): 899.

Klepzig, H. "Die konservative Therapie der Angina Pectoris." *Die Medizinische Welt* 24 (1973): 1926–1928.

Knightley, P., et al. *Suffer the Children: The Story of Thalidomide.* London: Viking Press, 1979.

Kohn, L., J. Corrigan, and M. Donaldson, eds. *To Err Is Human: Building a Safer Health System.* Washington, D.C.: Institute of Medicine, 2000.

Kolata, G. "Unorthodox Trials of AIDS Drugs Are Allowed by FDA." *New York Times*, 9 March 1990, A1.

Koll, W. "Fragen der experiementellen Teratologie im Rahmen der Arzneimittelprüfung." *Drug Research* 16 (1966): 1251–63.

———. "Dringende Bitte." February 1967. Reprinted in *Arzneimittelgesetzgebung, Arzneimittelprüfung, Arzneimittelbeobachtung in der Bundesrepublik Deutschland*, ed. Bundesärztekammer, 93–94. Köln: Duetsche Ärzte-Verlag.

Kollek, R. "Neue Kriterien für die Abschätzung des Risikos." In *Gentechnik—Wer kontrolliert die Industrie?*, ed. M. Thurau. Frankfurt am Main: Fischer Verlag, 1989.

Koller, S. "Über Möglichkeit und Wirksamkeit eines Beobachtungs- und Warnsystems zur frühzeitigen Erkennung gefährlicher Nebenwirkungen von Medikamenten." *Deutsches Ärzteblatt* (11 January 1964): 59–67.

Kramer, L. "The FDA's Callous Response to AIDS." *New York Times*, 23 March 1987, A19.

———. *The Destiny of Me.* New York: Penguin Books, 1993.

"Krebstherapie mit Interleukin-2 noch zu optimieren." *Pharmazeutische Zeitung* 135 (1990): 1116–17.

Kupec, I. "FDA Advisory Committee to Discuss Various AIDS Treatments." *Note to Correspondents*, 2 February 1996. ⟨http://www.fda.gov⟩. February 2002.

———. "FDA Grants Accelerated Approval to Third Protease Inhibitor to Treat HIV." *Press Release*, 14 March 1996. ⟨http://www.fda.gov⟩. February 2002.

Laar, J. "Versuche einer Harmonisierung der Arzneimittelgesetzgebung in der EWG." *Pharma Dialog* 24 (1973): 3–19.

Lamb, R. *American Chamber of Horrors: The Truth about Food and Drugs.* New York: Farrar & Rinehart, 1936.

Langbein, K., H. Weiss, and R. Werner. *Gesunde Geschäfte: Die Praktiken der Pharmaindustrie.* Köln: Kiepenheuer & Witsch, 1983.

Latour, B. "Give Me a Laboratory and I Will Raise the World." In *Science Observed*, ed. M. Mulkay and K. Knorr-Cetina, 141–70. London: Sage Publications, 1983.

——. *Science in Action: How to Follow Scientists and Engineers through Society*. Cambridge: Harvard University Press, 1987.

——. *The Pasteurization of France*. Cambridge: Harvard University Press, 1988.

——. *Pandora's Hope: Essays on the Reality of Science Studies*. Cambridge: Harvard University Press, 1999.

Latour B., and S. Woolgar. *Laboratory Life: The Construction of Scientific Facts*. Princeton: Princeton University Press, 1986.

Law, J., and M. Callon. "The Life and Death of an Aircraft: A Network Analysis of Technical Change." In *Shaping Technology/Building Society*, ed. W. Bijker and J. Law, 21–52. Cambridge: MIT Press, 1997.

Lazarou, J., et al. "Incidence of Adverse Drug Reactions in Hospitalized Patients." *JAMA* 279 (1998): 1200–1216.

Le Carré, J. *The Constant Gardener*. New York: Scribner, 2001.

Lear, J. "The Certification of Antibiotics." *Saturday Review*, 7 February 1959, 43–48.

——. "Taking the Miracle out of the Miracle Drugs." *Saturday Review*, 1 September 1962, 35–40.

——. "The Unfinished Story of Thalidomide." *Saturday Review*, 1 September 1962, 40–42.

Lehr, U. "Allgemeine Verwaltungsvorschrift zur Beobachtung, Sammlung, und Auswertung von Arzenimittelrisiken (Stufenplan) nach §63 des Arzneimittelgesetzes." *BAnz* 91 (16 May 1990): 2570.

Lenz, W. "Kindliche Missbildungen nach Medikament während der Gravidität." *Münchner medizinische Wochenschrift* 86 (1961): 2555–56.

——. "Thalidomide and Congenital Abnormalities." *Lancet* (6 January 1962): 45.

Lerner, B. *The Breast Cancer Wars: Hope, Fear, and the Pursuit of a Cure in Twentieth-Century America*. London: Oxford University Press, 2001.

Levi, J. "Unproven AIDS Therapies: The Food and Drug Administration and ddI." In *Biomedical Politics*, ed. K. Hanna, 9–37. Washington, D.C.: National Academy Press, 1991.

Lewin, T. "Families Sue Pfizer on Test of Antibiotic." *New York Times*, 30 August 2001.

Liebenau, J. *Medical Science and Medical Industry: The Formation of the American Pharmaceutical Industry*. Baltimore: Johns Hopkins University Press, 1987.

Lote, M., et al. "High-Dose Recombinant Interleukin-2 in the Treatment of Patients with Disseminated Cancer." *JAMA* 256 (1986): 3117–3124.

Löwy, I. *Between Bench and Bedside: Science, Healing, and Interleukin-2 in a Cancer Ward*. Cambridge: Harvard University Press, 1996.

Lueck, T. J. "Cetus Charting a Broad Course: Plans to Use Biotechnology in Many Fields." *New York Times*, 5 June 1981, 25.

Luhmann, N. *Soziale Systeme: Grundriß einer allgemeinen Theorie*. Frankfurt am Main: Suhrkamp, 1984.

Lunzer, F. "Trials of a Cancer Drug." *High Technology Business*, August 1988, 33–35.

Lydtin, H. "Die Bedeutung der ß-Blocker für die Hochdruckbehandlung." *Die Medizinische Welt* 26 (1975): 1487–92.

Maeder, T. *Adverse Reactions*. New York: Morrow Press, 1994.

Mahoney, T. *The Merchants of Life: An Account of the American Pharmaceutical Industry*. New York: Harper & Brothers, 1959.

Mainland, D. "Statistics in Clinical Research: Some General Principles." *Annals of the New York Academy of Sciences* 52 (1950): 922–30.

Mallard, A. "Compare, Standardize and Settle Agreement: On Some Usual Metrological Problems." *Social Studies of Science* 28 (1998): 571–601.

Marks, H. "Notes from the Underground: The Social Organization of Therapeutic Research." In *Grand Rounds: One Hundred Years of Internal Medicine*, ed. R. Maulitz and D. Long, 298–336. Philadelphia: University of Pennsylvania Press, 1988.

——. *The Progress of Experiment: Science and Therapeutic Reform in the United States, 1900–1990*. Cambridge: Cambridge University Press, 1997.

Marrus, M. "The Nuremberg Doctors' Trial in Historical Context." *Bulletin of the History of Medicine* 73 (1999): 106–23.

Martini, P. *Methodenlehre der therapeutischen Untersuchung*. Berlin: Verlag Julius Springer, 1932.

——. *Methodenlehre der Therapeutisch-Klinischen Forschung*. Berlin: Springer-Verlag, 1947.

——. "Einseitigkeit und Mitte in der Medizin." *Bonner Akademische Reden*. Bonn: Peter Haustein Verlag, 1954.

Matthews, J. R. *Quantification and the Quest for Medical Certainty*. Princeton: Princeton University Press, 1995.

Mbeki, T. "Speech at the Opening Session of the 13th International AIDS Conference," 9 July 2000. ⟨http://www.anc.org.za/ancdocs/history/mbeki/2000/tm0709.htm⟩. February 2002.

McBride, W. "Thalidomide and Congenital Abnormalities." *Lancet* (1961): 1358.

McFadyen, R. "Thalidomide in America: A Brush with Tragedy." *Clio Medica* 11 (1976): 79–93.

——. "The FDA's Regulation and Control of Antibiotics in the 1950s." *Bulletin of the History of Medicine* 53 (1979): 159–69.

"Menocil: Wie Zucker." *Der Spiegel*, 23 December 1968, 142–43.

Merck. "Livin' It Tools—Introduction," ⟨http://www.crixivan2.com/phys_new/livinitt/index.htm⟩. February 2002.

——. "Livin' It Tools—Personalized Treatment Planner." ⟨http://www.crixivan2.com.phys_new/livinitt/personal/index.htm⟩. February 2002.

——. "History of Crixivan—1995," ⟨http://www.crixivan2.com/phys_new/crixivan/1995.htm⟩. February 2002.

Merigan, T. "You Can Teach an Old Dog New Tricks: How AIDS Trials Are Pioneering New Strategies." *New England Journal of Medicine* 323 (1990): 1341–43.

Mines, S. *Pfizer: An Informal History*. New York: Pfizer, 1978.

Mintz, M. "Heroine of FDA Keeps Bad Drug off Market." *Washington Post*, 15 July 1962, A1.

Mintzes, B., et al. "Influence of Direct-to-Consumer Pharmaceutical Advertising and Patients' Requests on Prescribing Decisions." *British Medical Journal* 324 (2002): 278–79.

"Mißgeburten durch Tabletten? Alarmierender Verdacht eines Arztes gegen ein weitverbreitetes Medikament." *Welt am Sonntag*, 26 November 1961, S1.

Moertel, C. "On Lymphokines, Cytokines, and Breakthroughs." *JAMA* 256 (1986): 3141.

Monser, C. *Contergan/Thalidomid: Ein Unglück kommt selten allein*. Düsseldorf: Eggcup Verlag, 1993.

Moore, T. *Deadly Medicine*. New York: Simon & Schuster, 1995.

——. "FDA Earns Its Own Warning Label." *Boston Globe*, 2 April 2000.

Müller-Oerlinghausen, B. "Herstellerinteressen oder Patientenschutz?" *Deutsches Ärzteblatt* 92 (24 February 1995): 486.

Murswieck, A. *Die staatliche Kontrolle der Arzneimittelsicherheit in der Bundesrepublik und den USA*. Opladen: Westdeutscher Verlag, 1983.

National Kidney Cancer Association. "13 Steps to World Class Cancer Care" (brochure). Evanston: Kidney Cancer Association, n.d.

——. *We Have Kidney Cancer*. Evanston: Kidney Cancer Association, 1991.

Naughton, D. "Drug Lotteries Raise Questions: Some Experts Say System of Distribution May Be Unfair." *Washington Post*, 26 September 1995, Z14.

Neuhaus, G. "Versuche mit kranken Menschen—der kontrollierte klinische Versuch." In *Versuche mit Menschen*, ed. H. Helmchen and R. Winau, 108–32. Berlin: Walter de Gruyter, 1986.

"Nichtigkeit der Verordnung über die Herstellung von Arzneifertigwaren vom 11.Februar 1943." *Pharmazeutische Zeitung* 6 (1959): 143–44.

Nightingale, S. "International Harmonization: The ICH Process as a Model for Government and Industry Collaboration." *Swiss Pharma* 16 (1994): 59–63.

Nipperdey, T. *Germany from Napoleon to Bismarck, 1800–1866*. Princeton: Princeton University Press, 1996.

Nowak, R. "AIDS Researchers, Activists Fight Crisis in Clinical Trials." *Science* 269 (1995): 1666–67.

Nutley, C. "The Value and Benefits of ICH to Industry." ICH White Paper (January 2002). ⟨http://www.ifpma.org/ich1.html⟩. April 2003.

Office of Technology Assessment. "Product Liability and the Pharmaceutical Industry." In *Pharmaceutical R&D: Costs, Risks and Rewards*. Washington, D.C.: Government Printing Office, 1993.

Oldham, F. K., F. O. Kelsey, and E. M. K. Geiling. *Essentials of Pharmacology*. Philadelphia: J. B. Lippincott, 1947.

Oncologic Drugs Advisory Committee, Meeting # 55, Holiday Inn, Bethesda, Md., 19 December 1997.

Patrias, K., R. L. Gordner, and S. C. Groft. *Thalidomide: Potential Benefits and Risks [Bibliography Online]*. ⟨http://www.nlm.nih.gov/pubs/resources.html⟩. April 2002.

"Paul-Martini-Preis für Interleukin-2." *Pharmazeutische Zeitung* 134 (1989): 1971–72.

Payer, L. *Medicine and Culture*. New York: Henry Holt, 1996.

Peltzman, S. *Regulation of Pharmaceutical Innovation: The 1962 Amendments*. Washington, D.C.: American Enterprise Institute, 1974.

Pharmaceutical Research and Manufacturers of America. *Annual Report, 2000*. Washington, D.C.: PhRMA, 2000.

———. *Pharmaceutical Industry Profile 2000*. Washington, D.C.: PhRMA, 2000.

———. *Why Do Prescription Drugs Cost So Much?* Washington, D.C.: PhRMA, 2000.

———. *Pharmaceutical Industry Profile 2002*. Washington, D.C.: PhRMA, 2002.

———. *Pharmaceutical Industry Profile 2003*. Washington, D.C.: PhRMA, 2003.

"Pharma-Industrie warnt vor Bürokratismus auf dem Arzneimittelmarkt." *Deutsches Ärzteblatt*, 13 June 1974, 1805–06.

Pinch, T. J. "'Testing—One, Two, Three . . . Testing!': Toward a Sociology of Testing." *Science, Technology and Human Values* 18 (1993): 25–41.

Platzer, E. "Biologische Mediatoren in der Medizin." *Deutsches Ärzteblatt* 83 (1986): 3201–03.

Pollack, A., "Drug Makers Wrestle with World's New Rules." *New York Times*, 21 October 2001, A1.

Porter, T. *Trust in Numbers: The Pursuit of Objectivity in Science and Public Life*. Princeton: Princeton University Press, 1995.

"Präparate-kombinations günstig bei Angina Pectoris." *Deutsches Ärzteblatt* 49 (7 December 1968): 2823.

Price, D. K. *The Scientific Estate*. Cambridge: Harvard University Press, 1967.

Proctor, R. *Racial Hygiene: Medicine under the Nazis*. Cambridge: Harvard University Press, 1988.

Pross, C. "Introduction." In *Cleansing the Fatherland: Nazi Medicine and Racial Hygiene*, ed. G. Aly, P. Chroust, and C. Pross, 1–21. Baltimore: Johns Hopkins University Press, 1994.

"Protease Inhibitors May Increase Blood Glucose in HIV Patients." *FDA Medical Bulletin* 27 (Summer 1997).

Putnam, R. *Bowling Alone: The Collapse and Revival of American Community.* New York: Simon & Schuster, 2000.

Rabinow, P. *Making PCR: A Story of Biotechnology.* Chicago: University of Chicago Press, 1996.

"Der Regierungsentwurf des Arzneimittelgesetzes." *Die Pharmazeutische Industrie* 20 (1958): 421–22.

Reid, D. "Statistics in Clinical Research." *Annals of the New York Academy of Sciences* 52 (1950): 931.

Rhein-Pharma. *Dociton.* Frankfurt: Rhein-Pharma, 1965.

Richards, E. *Vitamin C and Cancer: Medicine or Politics?* New York: St. Martin's Press, 1991.

Ridder, P. *Im Spiegel der Arznei.* Stuttgart: S. Hirzel, 1990.

Riederer, J., and A. Lauer. "Nochmals die Stopverordnung." *Pharmazeutische Zeitung* 87 (1951): 382–85.

Riess, C. *Joseph Goebbels: Eine Biographie.* Baden-Baden: Dreieck Verlag, 1950.

Rosenberg, S. "Clinical Immunotherapy Studies in the Surgery Branch of the U.S. National Cancer Institute: Brief Review." *Cancer Treatment Review* 16 (1989): Suppl. A, 115–21.

Rosenberg, S., et al. "Experience with the Use of High-Dose Interleukin-2 in the Treatment of 652 Cancer Patients." *Annals of Surgery* 210 (1989): 474–85.

Rosenberg, S., and J. Barry. *Transformed Cell: Unlocking the Mysteries of Cancer.* New York: Avon Books, 1992.

Rosenbrock, R. *AIDS: Questions and Lessons for Public Health.* Berlin: Wissenschaftszentrum Berlin, 1992.

Rosenthal, M., et al. "Promotion of Prescription Drugs to Consumers." *New England Journal of Medicine* 346 (2002): 498–505.

Ross, O. "Use of Controls in Medical Research." *JAMA* 145 (1951): 72–75.

Rossi, A., and D. Knapp. "Discovery of New Adverse Drug Reactions: A Review of the Food and Drug Administration's Spontaneous Reporting System." *JAMA* 252 (1984): 1030–33.

Rueschemeyer, D. *Lawyers and Their Society: A Comparative Study of the Legal Profession in Germany and the United States.* Cambridge: Harvard University Press, 1973.

Sagar, A., A. Daemmrich, and M. Ashiya. "The Tragedy of the Commoners: Biotechnology and Its Publics." *Nature Biotechnology* 18 (January 2000): 2–4.

Salmen, A., ed. *ACT-UP: Feuer unterm Arsch.* Berlin: Deutsche AIDS-Hilfe, 1991.

Sander, A. "Positionspapier des Bundesverbandes der Pharmazeutischen Industrie." *Die Pharmzeutische Industrie* 51 (1989): 386–93.

Scheler, M. *Problems of a Sociology of Knowledge.* London: Routledge, 1980.

Schmidt, C. "Monitoring Research Overseas." *Modern Drug Discovery* (February 2001): 25–26.

Scott, J. C. *Seeing Like a State: How Certain Schemes to Improve the Human Condition Have Failed.* New Haven: Yale University Press, 1998.

Shapin, S. *A Social History of Truth: Civility and Science in Seventeenth-Century England.* Chicago: University of Chicago Press, 1994.

Shapiro, A., and E. Shapiro. *The Powerful Placebo: From Ancient Priest to Modern Physician.* Baltimore: Johns Hopkins University Press, 1997.

Shilts, R. *And the Band Played On: Politics, People, and the AIDS Epidemic.* New York: St. Martin's Press, 1987.

Sills, J., et al. "Postmarketing Reporting of Adverse Drug Reactions to the FDA: An Overview of the 1985 FDA Guideline." *Drug Information Journal* 20 (1986): 151–56.

Silverman, W. A., and I. Chalmers. "Sir Austin Bradford Hill: An Appreciation." *Controlled Clinical Trials* 13 (1992): 100–105.

Sinclair, U. *The Jungle.* New York: Doubleday, Page & Co., 1906.

Sjöström, H., and R. Nilsson. *Thalidomide and the Power of the Drug Companies.* Harmondsworth: Penguin Books, 1972.

Slutsker, G. "Look Before You Speak." *Forbes* 142 (26 December 1988): 116–17.

Smith, B. L. R. *American Science Policy since World War II.* Washington, D.C.: Brookings Institution, 1990.

Smith, R., and B. Wynne. *Expert Evidence: Interpreting Science in the Law.* New York: Routledge, 1989.

Soffer, A. "The Practitioner's Role in Detection of Adverse Drug Reactions." *Archives of Internal Medicine* 145 (1985): 232–33.

Speaker, S. "From 'Happiness Pills' to 'National Nightmare': Changing Cultural Assessment of Minor Tranquilizers in America, 1955–1980." *Journal of the History of Medicine and Allied Sciences* 52 (1997): 338–76.

Stapel, U. *Die Arzneimittelgesetze 1961 und 1976.* Stuttgart: Deutscher Apotheker Verlag, 1988.

Starr, P. *The Social Transformation of American Medicine.* New York: Basic Books, 1982.

Steinbach. "Bekanntmachung einer Empfehlung über die Mindestanforderungen an die pharmakologisch-toxicologische Prüfung als Voraussetzung für den Beginn der klinischen Prüfung von Arzneimitteln gegen HIV-Infektionen und AIDS bei Menschen." *Pharmazeutische Zeitung* 136 (1991): 3815.

Steinmetz, H. "Rekombinantes Interleukin-2." *Deutsche Apotheker Zeitung* 130 (1990): 2483–2484.

Stephens, T., and R. Brynner. *Dark Remedy: The Impact of Thalidomide and Its Revival as a Vital Medicine.* Cambridge, 2001.

Stigler, G. "The Theory of Economic Regulation." *Bell Journal of Economics and Management Science* 5 (1974): 337–52.

Stockhausen, J. "Erfassen, Sammeln und Auswerten von Arzneimittel-Nebenwirkungen." *Deutsches Ärzteblatt* (19 August 1971): 2326–2328.

Stokes, R. *Divide and Prosper: The Heirs of I. G. Farben under Allied Authority, 1945–1951.* Berkeley: University of California Press, 1988.

Stolberg, S. "The Boom in Medications Brings Rise in Fatal Risks." *New York Times,* 3 June 1999, A1, A18.

———. "Faulty Warning Labels Add to Risk in Prescription Drugs." *New York Times,* 4 June 1999, A23.

Stone, B. "How AIDS Has Changed FDA." *FDA Consumer* (February 1990): 14–17.

Streeck, W. "Between Pluralism and Corporatism: German Business Associations and the State." *Journal of Public Policy* 3 (1983): 265–84.

Sturm, A. "Mitteilungen des Vorstandes der Deutschen Gesellschaft für innere Medizin zur Aufstellung von Richtlinien für die klinische Prüfung von Arzneimitteln." *Klinische Wochenschrift* 43 (1965): 698–700.

Sullivan, A. "Pro Pharma." *New York Times Magazine,* 29 October 2000, 21–22.

"The Suspect and the Innocent." *JAMA* 196 (2 May 1966): 160.

Swann, J. "Sure Cure: Public Policy on Drug Efficacy before 1962." In *The Inside Story of Medicines,* ed. G. Higby and E. Stroud, 223–61. Madison: American Institute of the History of Pharmacy, 1997.

Task Force on Risk Management. *Managing the Risks from Medical Product Use: Creating a Risk Management Framework.* Rockville, Md.: U.S. Department of Health and Human Services, 1999.

Taussig, H. "A Study of the German Outbreak of Phocomelia." *JAMA* 180 (30 June 1962): 1106–14.

Teitelman, R. *Gene Dreams: Wall Street, Academia and the Rise of Biotechnology.* New York: Basic Books, 1987.

Temin, P. *Taking Your Medicine: Drug Regulation in the United States.* Cambridge: Harvard University Press, 1980.

"Terramycin, ein neues Antibiotikum." *Neue Medizinische Welt*, 2 September 1950, 1177.

Thayer, A. "Major Drug Firms Eke Out Increases." *Chemical and Engineering News*, 17 March 2003, 13–14.

Timmermans, S., and M. Berg. "Standardization in Action: Achieving Local Universality through Medical Protocols." *Social Studies of Science* 27 (1997): 273–305.

Timmermans, S., and V. Leiter. "The Redemption of Thalidomide: Standardizing the Risk of Birth Defects." *Social Studies of Science* 30 (2000): 41–71.

Überla, K. "Perspekitven der Erfassung und Bewertung unerwünschter Arzneimittelwirkungen." In *Arzneimittelsicherheit*, ed. P. Grosdanoff et al., 57–59. München: MMV Medizin Verlag, 1983.

United Nations–World Health Organization Working Group on Global HIV / AIDS. *Epidemiological Fact Sheets on HIV / AIDS and Sexually Transmitted Infections*. Geneva: UNAIDS / WHO, 2002.

U.S. Congress. "An Act for Preventing the Manufacture, Sale or Transportation of Adulterated or Misbranded or Poisonous or Deleterious Foods, Drugs, Medicines, and Liquors." 59th Cong., 1st sess. (30 June 1906), 34 U.S. Statutes 768.

——. "Federal Food, Drug, and Cosmetic Act." 75th Cong., 2nd sess. (25 June 1938). Washington, D.C.: Government Printing Office, 1938.

——. Senate. Judiciary Committee. Subcommittee on Antitrust and Monopoly. *Administered Prices*. 26 vols. Washington, D.C.: Government Printing Office, 1959–60.

——. Senate. Committee on Labor and Public Welfare. *Regulation of New Drug R&D by the Food and Drug Administration*. 93rd Cong., 2d sess. Washington, D.C.: Government Printing Office, 1974.

U.S. Department of Health, Education, and Welfare. "Doctor: Report Drug Reactions!" Leaflet No. 14, May 1965.

Verband Forschender Arzneimittelhersteller. *Statistics 2002: Die Arzneimittelindustrie in Deutschland*. Berlin: VFA, 2003.

Vogel, D. *National Styles of Regulation: Environmental Policy in Great Britain and the United States*. Ithaca: Cornell University Press, 1986.

von Beyme, K. "The Power Structure in the Federal Republic of Germany." In *Contemporary Germany: Politics & Culture*, ed. C. Burdick, H. Jacobsen, and W. Kudszus, 77–106. Boulder: Westview Press, 1984.

von Blanc, U. "Herstellung neuer Spezialitäten verboten!" *Die Pharmazeutische Industrie* 13 (1951): 33–36.

Vos, R. *Drugs Looking for Diseases: Innovative Research and the Development of the Beta Blockers and Calcium Antagonists*. Boston: Kluwer Academic Publishers, 1991.

Wardell, W., and L. Lasagna. "The 'Drug Lag' and American Therapeutics: An International Comparison." Talk presented at the Fifth International Congress of Pharmacology, 26 July 1972.

——. "Introduction of New Therapeutic Drugs in the United States and Great Britain: An International Comparison." *Clinical Pharmacology and Therapeutics* 14 (1973): 773–90.

——. *Regulation and Drug Development*. Washington, D.C.: American Enterprise Institute, 1975.

"A War over Drugs and Patents." *Economist*, 10 March 2001, 43–44.

Weindling, P. "The Origins of Informed Consent: The International Scientific Commission on Medical War Crimes, and the Nuremberg Code." *Bulletin of the History of Medicine* 75 (2001): 37–71.

Weingart, P., J. Kroll, and K. Bayertz. *Rasse, Blut und Gene: Geschichte der Eugenik und Rassenhygiene in Deutschland*. Frankfurt am Main: Suhrkamp Verlag, 1988.

Wenzel, D., and K. Wenzel. *Der Contergan-Prozeß (I): Verursachte Thalidomid Nervenschäden und Mißbildungen?* Benshein-Auerbach: Pressebüro Theilacker, 1968.

Westhoff, J. "Der Seehofer Skandal." *Pharmazeutische Zeitung* 138 (28 October 1993): 3444.

"Who Will Build Our Biodefenses?" *Economist*, 1 February 2003, 51–52.

Wiedebach, A. "Totale Phokomelie." *Zentralblatt für Gynäekologie* 81 (1959): 2048.

Wiener, J. B. "Managing the Iatrogenic Risks of Risk Management." *Risk: Health Safety & Environment* 39 (Winter 1998): 39–82.

Will, A. "Geheimniskrämerie bei der neuen europäischen Zulassungsbehörde." *BUKO Pharma-Brief*, May / June 1996, 1.

Willman, D. "Physician Who Opposes Rezulin Is Threatened by FDA with Dismissal." *Los Angeles Times*, 17 March 2001.

Winkle, W. V., R. Harwick, H. O. Calvery, and A. Smith. "Laboratory and Clinical Appraisal of New Drugs." *JAMA* 126 (1944): 956–61.

Wood, A., C. M. Stein, and R. Woosley. "Making Medicines Safer—The Need for an Independent Drug Safety Board." *New England Journal of Medicine* 339 (1998): 1851–54.

Yoshioka, A. "Streptomycin, 1946: British Central Administration of Supplies of a New Drug of American Origin with Special Reference to Clinical Trials in Tuberculosis." Ph.D. diss., Imperial College, 1998.

Young, J. H. *The Medical Messiahs: A Social History of Health Quackery in Twentieth-Century America.* Princeton: Princeton University Press, 1967.

———. *Pure Food: Securing the Federal Food and Drugs Act of 1906.* Princeton: Princeton University Press, 1989.

Young, R., and M. Surrusco. *Rx R&D Myths: The Case against the Drug Industry's R&D "Scare Card."* Washington, D.C.: Public Citizen, 2001.

"Zweites Gesetz zur Änderung des Arzneimittelgesetzes vom Bundestag verabschiedet." *Pharmazeutische Zeitung*, 7 May 1964, 670–76.

Index

Abbott Laboratories, 9, 104
Accelerated approval, 91
Adrenaline, 70
Adverse drug reactions. *See* Side effects
Advisory committees: FDA's use of, 27–28; in
    Germany, 42, 94; Cardiovascular Advisory
    Committee, 75–77; Biological Response Mod-
    ifiers Advisory Committee, 86–91; politics
    and, 89; Antiviral Drugs Advisory Commit-
    tee, 105–9
AIDS: politics and, 2–3; activists, 14, 30–32, 97–
    100, 105, 107, 113, 137; in Germany, 42–44, 96;
    AIDS Clinical Trials Group, 98; treatment of,
    103–11
AIDS-Beirat, 44, 101–2
AIDS Coalition to Unleash Power (ACT UP), 30–
    31, 44, 100, 105
AIDS-Hilfe, Deutsche, 43, 101
Alderin, 71
Alternative medicine, 41
American Cyanamid, 55
American Medical Association (AMA), 14, 119–25,
    132, 134, 136, 149, 155
Amyl Nitrates, 70, 72, 73
Angina pectoris, 69–71, 73, 74–77
Anthrax, 2–3
Antibiotics, 25, 37, 51, 55, 60, 69, 121, 130
Aplastic anemia, 121, 130
Arrhythmia, 74, 145
Arzneimittelinformationsdienst, 128
Arzneimittelinstitut, 142
Arzneimittelkommission der deutschen
    Ärzteschaft (AkdÄ), 39, 72–74, 117, 119, 126–
    32, 136, 141–47, 149, 155
Arzneiverordnungen, 126, 127
Aureomycin, 55
Aventis, 9

Ayerst, 74–77
AZT, 31–32, 44, 97, 100–110 passim

Barbiturates, 61
Barr, David, 100
BASF, 9, 92
Baycol, 140
Bayer, 2–3
Beecher, Henry, 68
Behringwerke, 92
Bendectin, 8
Beta-blockers, 29, 69–77
Bieter, Raymond, 67
Biotechnology, 83–86, 91–92
Black, James, 70
Boehringer Ingelheim, 58–59
Boston Globe, 91
British Medical Journal, 67
Brussels, 58
Büchner, Georg, 168 (n. 18)
BUKO-Pharmakampagne, 110
Bundesärztekammer (BÄK), 10, 36–53 passim, 72,
    74, 125–28, 132. *See also* Arzneimittelkommis-
    sion der deutschen Ärzteschaft
Bundesgesundheitsamt (BGA), 37–46 passim, 62,
    71, 73, 79, 83, 92–94, 103, 131, 133, 141–45
Bundesinstitut für Arzneimittel- und Medizin-
    produkte (BfArM), 11, 44, 117, 133, 145–47, 149
Bundeskanzler, 7
Bundesrat, 7
Bundestag, 7, 36–44 passim, 131, 133, 156
Bush, George W., 2
Business Week, 89

Camp, Rob, 107
Cancer, 81, 97–99, 113
Capillary leak syndrome, 85, 93, 95

Case studies: overview, 17, 154–55, 166
Cetus, 84–87, 92
"Chamber of horrors," 22
Chemie Grünenthal, 26, 61–63
Chinidin, 145
Chiron, 87–91, 93
Chloramphenicol, 121, 127, 130, 131
Chloromycetin, 55
Cilag, 130
Ciproflaxin, 2
Clinical pharmacology, 50, 66, 82
Clinical trials: contestation and debate over, 12–13, 77–78; in U.S. and Germany, 17–18, 42, 48–50, 72, 96, 159; methods for carrying out, 48–54, 56, 58, 60, 62, 64, 68, 86, 87, 90, 97–101, 158; role of statistics in, 51–54, 78–80; broader medical role of, 101, 148, 154–55. *See also* Standardization: of clinical trials
Committee on Adverse Reactions (AMA Council on Drugs), 121–25
Committee on Blood Dyscrasias (AMA Council on Drugs), 121, 125
Commission on Proprietary Medicinal Products (CPMP), 110–11
Committee on the Safety of Medicines (U.K.), 73
Contergan, 38–40, 61–65; trial, 63–65. *See also* Thalidomide
Copeland, Royal, 22, 23
Cordichin, 145–47
Council on Drugs (AMA), 28, 117, 121–25, 128, 132, 133, 134, 149, 155
Council on Pharmacy and Chemistry (AMA), 24, 120–21
Cox, Spencer, 107
Crixivan, 103–14

Dalkon Shield, 8
Deutsches Ärzteblatt, 92, 127, 128
Diabetes, 109, 140
DiMasi, Joseph, 161
Disease-based organizations. *See* Patients
Dociton, 71–74. *See also* Propranolol
Double-blind trials, 51, 52, 54, 69, 74–76. *See also* Clinical trials
Dowling, Harry, 121
Drug Experience Report, 124–25, 134–35, 138
Drug lag, 29–30, 44
Drug prices, 1–3, 25, 91, 161
Dukes, M. N. G., 162

Eastern Cooperative Oncology Group (ECOG), 87–89, 93

Efficacy, 1–3, 6, 10–12, 24–49 passim, 63, 66, 69, 82, 159
Encaid, 140
Epivir, 105, 109
Epstein, Steven, 100
Eurocetus, 92–95
European Agency for the Evaluation of Medicinal Products (EMEA), 82–83, 103, 111–14, 157, 158
European AIDS Treatment Group, 107
European Commission, 40, 157
European Federation of Pharmaceutical Industries and Associations, 157
European Public Assessment Report (EPAR), 110–13
European Union, 45, 80

Federal Chamber of Physicians. *See* Bundesärztekammer
Federal Health Office. *See* Bundesgesundheitsamt
Food and Drug Administration (FDA): impact of on medical profession, 10; and labeling controls, 24–25, 77; Bureau of Medicine, 26; criticism of by activists, 30–32, 97–99; Cancer Liaison Program, 98–99; monitoring of side effects by, 117, 119, 124–25, 132, 149, 155; institutional affiliation of, 169 (n. 5)
Food and drug laws (U.S.): 1906 Pure Food and Drug Law, 21–22; 1938 amendments, 23–24, 52, 58, 67; 1962 Kefauver-Harris Amendments, 27–30, 69, 74, 124; 1983 Orphan Drug Act, 30; parallel track review, 32, 98; treatment investigational new drug regulations, 32, 98; Modernization Act, 32–33; Prescription Drug User Fee Act, 32–33; "Single Patient Investigational New Drug Applications," 99
Fortune, 84–85
Frenkel, Horst
Friedman, Milton, 29

Gallo, Robert, 83–84
Gay Men's Health Crisis, 30
German Democratic Republic, 6
German Drug Commission. *See* Arzneimittel-kommission der deutschen Ärzteschaft
German drug laws: 1872 precursor, 34; Stop-Verordnung, 35–37; 1961 law, 38–39; 1964 law, 39; 1976 law, 41–42, 101, 141, 142; 1989 and 1990 amendments, 44; 1986 amendments, 143
German government: overview, 6–8; Federal Constitutional Court, 8, 37; Second Empire, 34; Interior Ministry, 36–37, 59, 60, 79

German Pharmacology Society, 39
German Society for Internal Medicine, 39
Goebbels, Joseph, 35
Gold, Harry, 52
Grabowski, Henry, 29
Grinberg, Linda, 107
Grundgesetz, 7

Harmonization, x, 3, 149, 155, 158, 162. *See also* International harmonization
Harris, Oren, 27
Heart disease, 69–71, 74–75
Heberden, William, 70
Heinzler, Franz, 63–64, 65, 67
Henneberg, Georg, 142
Hepatitis-B, 92
Heubner, Wolfgang, 63
Hill, Austin Bradford, 51–52, 60, 80
HIV. *See* AIDS
Hoechst, 9, 92
Hoffman-LaRoche, 100, 104
Hypertension, 69–71, 74–77, 130

I. G. Farben, 22
Imperial Chemical Industries (ICI), 70, 73, 74
Inderal, 74–77. *See also* Propranolol
Indinavir, 17, 48, 81. *See also* Crixivan
Institute for Drugs. *See* Arzneimittelinstitut
Institute of Medicine, 140
Insurance, 4
Interferon-alpha, 93
Interleukin-2 (IL-2), 17, 48, 81, 83–95; subcutaneous administration of, 93
International harmonization: International Conference on Harmonisation of Technical Requirements for Registration of Pharmaceuticals for Human Use (ICH), 3, 157–60; European participation in, 15; U.S. participation in, 15, 157
Interpretive flexibility, 12

Jasanoff, Sheila, 13, 27
Jenner, Edward, 51
Joint Commission on Accreditation of Hospitals, 121
Journal of the American Medical Association (JAMA), 55, 85, 120–23

Kattus, Albert, 75
Kefauver, Estes, 25–28, 141
Kelsey, Frances, 26–28, 66–68
Kennedy, John F., 27

Kessler, David, 108, 137–38
Kevadon. *See* Thalidomide
Kidney cancer, 86, 87, 94, 99
Kidney stones, 106, 107
King, Ernest, 57
Knoll, 146
Kramer, Larry, 30, 100

Lancet, 62, 73
Lasagna, Louis, 29
Latour, Bruno, 79, 118, 136
Lear, John, 27, 57, 68
Le Carre, John, 152
Lenz, Widukind, 61–62, 67, 68
Leukemia, 87
Levin, Jules, 107
Lind, James, 50–51
Lydtin, Helmut, 73

Marks, Harry, 23, 24, 54, 80
Martini, Paul, 51–54, 56, 60, 63–65
Massengill, S. E., 23
Mayo Clinic, 85
Mbeki, Thado, 103
McDermott, Walsh, 55
McKeen, John, 55
Medical Research Council, 51
MEDWatch, 137–40
Menocil, 130, 131
Merck, 103–11
Merrell, William S., Inc., 26–27, 66–68
Metastatic melanoma, 90
Mielke, Fred, 53
Minden Pharma, 146
Ministry of Health, Labor and Welfare (Japan), 157
Mitscherlich, Alexander, 53
Moertel, Charles, 85, 88
Müller-Oerlinghausen, Bruno, 146–47

Nader, Ralph, 161
National AIDS Treatment Advocacy Project, 107
National Breast Cancer Coalition, 30
National Cancer Institute (NCI), 83, 85, 87, 92, 93
National Formulary (NF), 21–22, 28
National Institute of Allergy and Infectious Diseases, 98
National Institutes of Health (NIH), 30, 31, 87, 97, 100, 161
National Kidney Cancer Association (NKCA), 98–99
National Organization for Rare Disorders, 30

National Socialism: impact of, 7, 53; drug regulation and, 35–36; medical practice and profession under, 35–36, 54, 126–27

Nebuchadnezzar II, 50

Network theory, 11–12

Newsweek, 84–85

Nitroglycerin, 70, 75, 77

Non-Governmental Organizations (NGOs): patients' groups, 10

Norvir, 104

Novartis, 69

Nuremberg: physicians' trial, 53; code, 54

Parke-Davis, 55

Pasteur, Louis, 50

Patents, 2, 25

Patients: asserting own voices and authority, 3, 6, 14, 17, 30–34, 45–47, 80, 81–83, 97–99, 107, 113, 133, 137, 141, 156, 162; spoken for by physicians or government, 4, 10–11, 17, 20–21, 24, 29, 37, 111, 125, 156; as "guinea pigs," 16, 27, 141; as cases, 49, 53, 56; social and political standing of, 117, 119–20, 153–55, 160

Payer, Lynn, 70

Peltzman, Samuel, 29

Penicillin, 24, 55, 60

Peripheral neuritis, 61, 67

Pfizer, 55–58, 152

Pharmaceutical industry: data on, 2, 9; overview, 8–10; marketing practices, 24–25, 68–69; innovation in, 29; German, 36–37, 38, 94; use of clinical trials by, 49

Pharmaceutical Manufacturers Association (Japan), 157

Pharmaceutical politics, 1–3

Pharmaceutical Research and Manufacturers of America, 157

Pharmacovigilance, 116–17. *See also* Side effects

Phenobarbital, 127

Phocomelia, 60

Placebo, 51, 53, 54, 56, 64, 69, 74, 76, 82, 97

Policy: science and medicine, 13–15

Polymerase chain reaction (PCR), 87

Porter, Ted, 79

Practolol, 29, 73, 74

Project Inform, 30, 105, 107

Proleukin, 84–95, 113–14. *See also* Interleukin-2

Propranolol, 17, 29, 48, 70, 73, 74–77, 91

Propulsid, 140

Public Citizen, 161

Quantification. *See* Clinical trials: role of statistics in

Race: and side effects, 118, 121, 123, 134, 138

Randomization, 51, 56, 58. *See also* Clinical trials: methods for carrying out

Reagan, Ronald, 84

Redux, 140

Regulation: precautionary, 13, 29, 54. *See also* Bundesgesundheitsamt; Bundesinstitut für Arzneimittel- und Medizinprodukte; Food and Drug Administration; Risk

Replication, 12

Rezulin, 140

Rhein-Pharma, 71

Rhône-Poulenc, 9

Risk, 13, 23, 46, 72, 113, 145, 149, 159, 160, 161, 162

Roosevelt, Theodore, 21

Rosenberg, Steven, 84, 87

Ross, Ortho, 56

Safety, 1–3, 6, 10–12, 23–49 passim, 69, 82, 159

Saquinavir, 100, 104

Saturday Review, 27, 57, 68

Schmidt, Alexander, 30

Seal of Acceptance Program, 120

Sedatives. *See* Thalidomide

Shapin, Steven, 156–57

Side effects: and data collection in U.S. and Germany, 18, 116–17; low incidence of with antibiotics, 60; and Thalidomide, 64, 66–67; and beta-blockers, 70, 78; and Proleukin, 88, 90, 93; and Crixivan, 106; registries of, 123–25, 127–29, 142–45; legislative responses to, 153–54

Silicon implants, 8

Sinclair, Upton, 21

Society for Internal Medicine (Germany), 126

Society for Pediatric Medicine (Germany), 62

Spiegel, Der, 63

Stadtlanders, 109

Standardization, 11–12, 160; of clinical trials, 3, 11, 24, 49–50, 67–68, 76, 78–80, 159, 160; of patients, 53, 68; of reports of adverse reactions, 119, 136, 148–50

Statistics and statisticians. *See* Clinical trials

Streptomycin, 51, 52, 55, 58

Stufenplan, 117, 141–47

Sulfa drugs, 60. *See also* Sulfanilamide

Sulfanilamide, 22–23, 32, 46

Sullivan, Andrew, 9

Surrogate endpoints, 98–99, 114

Tambocor, 140

Teitelman, Robert, 86

Terra Haute, Indiana, 55
Terramycin, 17, 48, 54–60
Testing and market: boundary between, 5–6, 20, 74, 156
Thalidomide, 17, 26–27, 29, 32, 45, 46, 48, 60–69; impact of, 127–28, 131, 134, 147
Therapeutic cultures: defined, 3–5, 151, 156–57; comparison of, 5–6, 47, 70, 78, 81, 99, 114–15, 116–17; and principal actors in medical policy, 11–12, 111; sites of impact, 16, 152–55; drug laws and, 20–21, 46; clinical trials and, 48–49, 72, 91; data collection under, 132–33, 137–38
Therapeutic reformers, 23, 45, 49, 52, 66
Translation of data, 119–20, 134–36
Treatment Action Group (TAG). See AIDS: activists

Überla, Karl, 142–43
U.S. government: overview, 6–8; Congress, 7; Senate, 7; Supreme Court, 8, 22; Department of Agriculture, 21; Senate Judiciary Committee, 25–26
United States Pharmacopoeia (USP), 21–22, 28

Verapamil, 145
Virchow, Rudolph, 168 (n. 18)
Vorlaender, Karl Otto, 64–65, 67, 68
Voss, Ralph, 61

Wardell, William, 29
Warner-Lambert, 140
Weimar Republic, 34
Welch, Henry, 57–58
Welt am Sonntag, 62
Wiener, Jonathan, 13
Wiley, Harvey, 21
Wirtschaftswunder, 36
World War II, 35–36, 52

Zidovudine. See AZT

Studies in Social Medicine

Nancy M. P. King, Gail E. Henderson, and Jane Stein, eds., *Beyond Regulations: Ethics in Human Subjects Research* (1999).

Laurie Zoloth, *Health Care and the Ethics of Encounter: A Jewish Discussion of Social Justice* (1999).

Susan M. Reverby, ed., *Tuskegee's Truths: Rethinking the Tuskegee Syphilis Study* (2000).

Beatrix Hoffman, *The Wages of Sickness: The Politics of Health Insurance in Progressive America* (2000).

Margarete Sandelowski, *Devices and Desires: Gender, Technology, and American Nursing* (2000).

Keith Wailoo, *Dying in the City of the Blues: Sickle Cell Anemia and the Politics of Race and Health* (2001).

Judith Andre, *Bioethics as Practice* (2002).

Chris Feudtner, *Bittersweet: Diabetes, Insulin, and the Transformation of Illness* (2003).

Ann Folwell Stanford, *Bodies in a Broken World: Women Novelists of Color and the Politics of Medicine* (2003).

Lawrence O. Gostin, *The AIDS Pandemic: Complacency, Injustice, and Unfulfilled Expectations* (2003).

Arthur A. Daemmrich, *Pharmacopolitics: Drug Regulation in the United States and Germany* (2004).